THE SILENT SPEAKER

The NIA (National Industrial Association) was one of the most powerful and wealthy organizations in America. Nero Wolfe couldn't care less. Then murder mingled with money, people began interpreting the group's initials as "Not Innocent Atall," and a delegation of millionaires—all of them suspects—convinced Nero (over $10,000 worth) to take a very active interest . . .

". . . NERO AND ARCHIE AT THEIR UPROARIOUS BEST."

—The New York Times

Books by Rex Stout

- THE SILENT SPEAKER
- TOO MANY WOMEN
- AND BE A VILLAIN
- THE SECOND CONFESSION
- TROUBLE IN TRIPLICATE
- CURTAINS FOR THREE
- IN THE BEST FAMILIES
- THREE DOORS TO DEATH
- MURDER BY THE BOOK
- PRISONER'S BASE
- TRIPLE JEOPARDY
- THE GOLDEN SPIDERS
- THE BLACK MOUNTAIN
- THREE MEN OUT
- BEFORE MIDNIGHT
- MIGHT AS WELL BE DEAD
- THREE WITNESSES
- IF DEATH EVER SLEPT
- THREE FOR THE CHAIR
- AND FOUR TO GO
- CHAMPAGNE FOR ONE
- PLOT IT YOURSELF
- THREE AT WOLFE'S DOOR
- TOO MANY CLIENTS
- THE FINAL DEDUCTION
- GAMBIT
- HOMICIDE TRINITY
- THE MOTHER HUNT
- A RIGHT TO DIE
- TRIO FOR BLUNT INSTRUMENTS
- THE DOORBELL RANG

Published by Bantam Books, Inc.

A NERO WOLFE NOVEL

THE SILENT SPEAKER

BY REX STOUT

BANTAM BOOKS · TORONTO · NEW YORK · LONDON

*This low-priced Bantam Book
has been completely reset in a type face
designed for easy reading, and was printed
from new plates. It contains the complete
text of the original hard-cover edition.*
NOT ONE WORD HAS BEEN OMITTED.

THE SILENT SPEAKER
*A Bantam Book / published by arrangement with
The Viking Press, Inc.*

PRINTING HISTORY
Viking edition published October 1946
Detective Book Club edition published December 1946
Bantam edition published October 1948
New Bantam edition published July 1958
2nd printing.......August 1967
3rd printing
4th printing

*The characters in this book are imaginary, and
resemblances to them, if any, borne by actual persons or
corpses are accidental and in some cases deplorable.*

Published simultaneously in the United States and Canada

---

*Bantam Books are published by Bantam Books, Inc., a subsidiary
of Grosset & Dunlap, Inc. Its trade-mark, consisting of the words
"Bantam Books" and the portrayal of a bantam, is registered in the
United States Patent Office and in other countries. Marca Registrada.
Bantam Books, Inc., 271 Madison Avenue, New York, N.Y. 10016.*

PRINTED IN THE UNITED STATES OF AMERICA

THE SILENT SPEAKER

1.

SEATED in his giant's chair behind his desk in his office, leaning back with his eyes half closed, Nero Wolfe muttered at me:

"It is an interesting fact that the members of the National Industrial Association who were at that dinner last evening represent, in the aggregate, assets of something like thirty billion dollars."

I slid the checkbook into place on top of the stack, closed the door of the safe, twirled the knob, and yawned on the way back to my desk.

"Yes, sir," I agreed with him. "It is also an interesting fact that the prehistoric Mound Builders left more traces of their work in Ohio than in any other state. In my boyhood days—"

"Shut up," Wolfe muttered.

I let it pass without any feeling of resentment, first because it was going on midnight and I was sleepy, and second because it was conceivable that there might be some connection between his interesting fact and our previous conversation, and that was not true of mine. We had been discussing the bank balance, the reserve against taxes, expectations as to bills and burdens, one of which was my salary, and related matters. The exchequer had not swung for the third strike, but neither had it knocked the ball out of the park.

After I had yawned three more times Wolfe spoke suddenly and decisively.

"Archie. Your notebook. Here are directions for tomorrow."

In two minutes he had me wide awake. When he had finished and I went upstairs to bed, the program for the morning was so active in my head that I tossed and turned for a full thirty seconds before sleep came.

2.

THAT was a Wednesday toward the end of the warmest March in the history of New York. Thursday it was more of the same, and I didn't even take a topcoat when I left the house on West Thirty-fifth Street and went to the garage for the car. I was fully armed, prepared for all contingencies. In my wallet was a supply of engraved cards reading:

ARCHIE GOODWIN

With Nero Wolfe
922 West 35th Street PRoctor 5-5000

And in the breast pocket of my coat, along with the routine cargo, was a special item just manufactured by me on the typewriter. It was on a printed Memo form and, after stating that it was FOR Nero Wolfe and FROM Archie Goodwin, it went on:

> *Okay from Inspector Cramer for inspection of the room at the Waldorf. Will report later by phone.*

At the right of the typing, scribbled in ink, also my work and worthy of admiration, were the initials LTC.

Since I had got an early start and the office of the Homicide Squad on Twentieth Street was less than a mile downtown, it was only a little after nine-thirty when I was admitted to an inside room and took a chair at the end of a crummy old desk. The man in the swivel chair, frowning at papers, had a big round red face, half-hidden gray eyes, and delicate little ears that stayed close to his skull. As I sat down he transferred the frown to me and grunted:

"I'm busy as hell." His eyes focused three inches below my chin. "What do you think it is, Easter?"

"I know of no law," I said stiffly, "against a man's buying a new shirt and tie. Anyhow, I'm in disguise as a detective. Sure you're busy, and I won't waste your time. I want to ask a favor, a big favor. Not for me, I'm quite aware that if I were trapped in a burning building you would yell for gasoline to toss on the flames, but on behalf of Nero Wolfe. He wants permission for me to inspect that room at the Waldorf where Cheney Boone was murdered Tuesday evening. Also maybe to take pictures."

Inspector Cramer stared at me, not at my new tie. "For God's sake," he said finally in bitter disgust. "As if this case wasn't enough of a mess already. All it needed to make it a carnival was Nero Wolfe, and by God here he is." He worked his jaw, regarding me sourly. "Who's your client?"

I shook my head. "I have no information about any client. As far as I know it's just Mr. Wolfe's scientific curiosity. He's interested in crime—"

"You heard me, who's your client?"

"No, sir," I said regretfully. "Rip me open, remove my heart for the laboratory, and you'll find inscribed on it—"

"Beat it," he grated, and dug into his papers.

I stood up. "Certainly, Inspector, I know you're busy. But Mr. Wolfe would greatly appreciate it if you'll give me permission to inspect—"

"Nuts." He didn't look up. "You don't need any permission to inspect and you know damn well you don't. We're all through up there and it's public premises. If what you're after is authority, it's the first time Wolfe ever bothered to ask for authority to do anything he wanted to do, and if I had time I'd try to figure out what the catch is, but I'm too busy. Beat it."

"Gosh," I said in a discouraged tone, starting for the door. "Suspicious. Always suspicious. What a way to live."

3.

In appearance, dress, and manner, Johnny Darst was about as far as you could get from the average idea of a hotel dick. He might have been taken for a vice-president of a trust company or a golf club steward. In a little room, more a cubbyhole than a room in size, he stood watching me deadpan while I looked over the topography, the angles, and the furniture, which consisted of a small table, a mirror, and a few chairs. Since Johnny was not a sap I didn't even try to give him the impression that I was doing something abstruse.

"What are you really after?" he asked gently.

"Nothing whatever," I told him. "I work for Nero Wolfe just as you work for the Waldorf, and he sent me here to take a look and here I am. The carpet's been changed?"

He nodded. "There was a little blood, not much, and the cops took some things."

"According to the paper there are four of these rooms, two on each side of the stage."

He nodded again. "Used as dressing rooms and resting rooms for performers. Not that you could call Cheney Boone a performer. He wanted a place to look over his speech and they sent him in here to be alone. The Grand Ballroom of the Waldorf is the best-equipped—"

"Sure," I said warmly. "You bet it is. They ought to pay you extra. Well, I'm a thousand times obliged."

"Got all you want?"

"Yep, I guess I've solved it."

"I could show you the exact spot where he was going to stand to deliver his speech if he had still been alive."

"Thanks a lot, but if I find I need that I'll come back."

He went with me down in the elevator and to the entrance, both of us understanding that the only private detectives hotels enjoy having around are the ones they hire. At the door he asked casually:

"Who's Wolfe working for?"

"There is never," I told him, "any question about that. He is working first, last, and all the time for Wolfe. Come to think of it, so am I. Boy, am I loyal."

4.

It was a quarter to eleven when I parked the car in Foley Square, entered the United States Court House, and took the elevator.

There were a dozen or more FBI men with whom Wolfe and I had had dealings during the war, when he was doing chores for the government and I was in G-2. It had been decided that for the present purpose G. G. Spero, being approximately three per cent less tight-lipped than the others, was the man, so it was to him I sent my card. In no time at all a clean efficient girl took me to a clean efficient room, and a clean efficient face, belonging to G. G. Spero of the FBI, was confronting me. We chinned a couple of minutes and then he asked heartily:

"Well, Major, what can we do for you?"

"Two little things," I replied. "First, quit calling me Major. I'm out of uniform, and besides, it stimulates my inferiority complex because I should have been a colonel. Second is a request from Nero Wolfe, sort of confidential. Of course he could have sent me to the Chief, or phoned him, but he didn't want to bother him about it. It's a little question about the Boone murder case. We've been told that the FBI is mixing in, and of course you don't ordinarily touch a local murder. Mr. Wolfe would like to know if there is something about the FBI angle that would make it undesirable for a private detective to take any interest."

Spero was still trying to look cordial, but training and habit were too much for him. He started to drum on the desk, realized what he was doing, and jerked his hand away. FBI men do not drum on desks.

"The Boone case," he said.

"That's right. The Cheney Boone case."

"Yes, certainly. Putting aside, for the moment, the FBI angle, what would Mr. Wolfe's angle be?"

He went at me and kept after me from forty different directions. I left half an hour later with what I had expected to leave with, nothing. The reliance on his three per cent under par in lip tightness was not for the sake of what he might tell me, but what he might tell about me.

5.

THE last number on the program proved to be the most complicated, chiefly because I was dealing with total strangers. I didn't know a soul connected with the National Industrial Association, and so had to start from scratch. The whole atmosphere, from the moment I entered the offices on the thirtieth floor of a building on Forty-first Street, made a bad impression on me. The reception room was too big, they had spent too much money on rugs, upholstery had been carried to extremes, and the girl at the desk, though not a bad specimen from the standpoint of design, had been connected up with a tube running from a refrigerating unit. She was so obviously congealed for good that there wasn't the slightest temptation to start thawing her out. With females between twenty and thirty, meeting a certain standard in contour and coloring, I do not believe in being distant, but I was with that one as I handed her a card and said I wanted to see Hattie Harding.

The hurdles I had to make, you might have thought Hattie Harding was the goddess of a temple and this was it, instead of merely the Assistant Director of Public Relations for the NIA, but I finally made the last jump and was taken in to her. Even she had space, rugs, and upholstery. Personally, she had quality, but the kind that arouses one or two of my most dangerous instincts, and I do not mean what some may think I mean. She was somewhere between twenty-six and forty-eight, tall, well put together, well dressed, and had skeptical, competent dark eyes which informed you with the first glance that they knew everything in the world.

"This is a pleasure," she declared, giving me a firm and not cold handshake. "To meet *the* Archie Goodwin, coming direct from *the* Nero Wolfe. Really a great pleasure. At least, I suppose you do? Come direct, I mean?"

I concealed my feelings. "On a beeline, Miss Harding. As the bee from the flower."

She laughed competently. "What! Not to the flower?"

I laughed back. We were chums. "I guess that's nearer the truth, at that, because I admit I've come to get a load of nectar. For Nero Wolfe. He thinks he needs a list of the members of the NIA who were at that dinner at the Waldorf Tuesday evening, and sent me here to get it. He has a copy of the printed list, but he needs to know who is on it that didn't come and who came that isn't on it. What do you think of my syntax?"

She didn't answer that, and she was through laughing. She asked, not as chum to chum, "Why don't we sit down?"

She moved toward a couple of chairs near a window, but I pretended not to notice and marched across to one for visitors at the end of her desk, so she would have to take her desk chair. The Memo from me to Wolfe, initialed for Inspector Cramer by me, was now in the side pocket of my coat, destined to be left on the floor of Miss Harding's office, and with the corner of her desk between us the operation would be simple.

"This is very interesting," she declared. "What does Mr. Wolfe want the list for?"

"Being honest," I smiled at her, "I can but tell you an honest lie. He wants to ask them for their autographs."

"I'm honest too," she smiled back. "Look, Mr. Goodwin. You understand of course that this affair is in the highest degree inconvenient for my employers. Our guest of the evening, our main speaker, the Director of the Bureau of Price Regulation, murdered right there just as the dinner was starting. I am in a perfectly terrible spot. Even if for the past ten years this office has done the best public relations job on record, which I am not claiming for it, all its efforts may have been destroyed by what happened there in ten seconds. There is no—"

"How do you know it happened in ten seconds?"

She blinked at me. "Why—it must—the way—"

"Not proven," I said conversationally. "He was hit four times on the head with the monkey wrench. Of course the blows could all have been struck within ten seconds. Or the murderer could have hit him once and knocked him unconscious, rested a while and then hit him again, rested some more and hit him the third—"

"What are you doing?" she snapped. "Just trying to see how objectionable you can be?"

"No, I'm demonstrating what a murder investigation is like. If you made that remark to the police, that it happened in ten seconds, you'd never hear the last of it. With me it goes in one ear and out the other, and anyhow I'm not interested, since I'm here only to get what Mr. Wolfe sent me for, and we'd greatly appreciate it if you would give us that list."

I was all set for quite a speech, but stopped on seeing her put both hands to her face, and I was thinking my lord she's going to weep with despair at the untimely end of public relations, but all she did was press the heels of her palms against her eyes and keep them there. It was the perfect moment to drop the Memo on the rug, so I did.

She kept her hands pressed to her eyes long enough for me to drop a whole flock of memos, but when she finally removed them the eyes still looked competent.

"I'm sorry," she said, "but I haven't slept for two nights and I'm a wreck. I'll have to ask you to go. There's to be another conference in Mr. Erskine's office about this awful business, it starts in ten minutes and I'll have to do myself for it, and anyway you know perfectly well I couldn't give you that list without approval from higher up, and besides if Mr. Wolfe is as intimate with the police as people say, why can't he get it from them? Talk about your syntax, look at the way I'm talking. Only one thing you might tell me, I sincerely hope you will, who has engaged Mr. Wolfe to work on this?"

I shook my head and got upright. "I'm in the same fix you are, Miss Harding. I can't do anything important, like answering a plain simple question, without approval from higher up. How about a bargain? I'll ask Mr. Wolfe if I may answer your question, and you ask Mr. Erskine if you may give me the list. Good luck at your conference."

We shook hands, and I crossed the rugs to the door without lingering, not caring to have her find the Memo in time to pick it up and hand it to me.

The midtown midday traffic being what it was, the short trip to West Thirty-fifth Street was a crawl all the way. I parked in front of the old stone house, owned by Nero Wolfe, that had been my home for over ten years, mounted the stoop, and tried to get myself in with my key, but found that the bolt was in and had to ring the bell. Fritz Brenner, cook, housekeeper, and groom of the chambers, came and opened up, and, informing him that the chances looked good for getting paid Saturday, I went down the hall to the office. Wolfe was seated behind his desk, reading a book. That was the only spot where he was ever really comfortable. There were other chairs in the house that had been made to order, for width and depth, with a guaranty for up to five hundred pounds—one in his room, one in the kitchen, one in the dining room, one in the plant rooms on the roof where the orchids were kept, and one there in the office, over by the two-foot globe and the book-shelves—but it was the one at his desk that nearly always got it, night and day.

As usual, he didn't lift an eye when I entered. Also as usual, I paid no attention to whether he was paying attention.

"The hooks are baited," I told him. "Probably at this very moment the radio stations are announcing that Nero Wolfe, the greatest living private detective when he feels like working, which isn't often, is wrapping up the Boone case. Shall I turn it on?"

He finished a paragraph, dog-eared a page, and put the book down. "No," he said. "It's time for lunch." He eyed me. "You must have been uncommonly transparent. Mr. Cramer has phoned. Mr. Travis of the FBI has phoned. Mr. Rohde of the Waldorf has phoned. It seemed likely that one or more of them would be coming here, so I had Fritz bolt the door."

That was all for the moment, or rather for the hour or more, since Fritz entered to announce lunch, which that day happened to consist of corn cakes with breaded fresh pork tenderloin, followed by corn cakes with a hot sauce of tomatoes and cheese, followed by corn cakes with honey. Fritz's timing with corn cakes was superb. At the precise instant, for example, that one of us finished with his eleventh, here came the twelfth straight from the griddle, and so on.

6.

I CALLED it Operation Payroll. That name for the preliminary project, the horning-in campaign, was not, I admit, strictly accurate. In addition to the salaries of Fritz Brenner, Charley the cleaning man, Theodore Horstmann the orchid tender, and me, the treasury had to provide for other items too numerous to mention. But on the principle of putting first things first, I called it Operation Payroll.

It was Friday morning before we caught the fish we were after. All that happened Thursday afternoon was a couple of unannounced visits, one from Cramer and one from G. G. Spero, and Wolfe had told me not to let them in, so they went away without crossing the sill. To show how sure I felt that the fish would sooner or later bite. I took the trouble Thursday afternoon and evening to get up a typed report of the Boone case as I knew it, from newspaper accounts and a talk I had had Wednesday with Sergeant Purley Stebbins. I've just read that report over again and decided not to copy it all down here but only hit the high spots.

Cheney Boone, Director of the government's Bureau of Price Regulation, had been invited to make the main speech at a dinner of the National Industrial Association on Tuesday evening at the Grand Ballroom of the Waldorf-Astoria. He had arrived at ten minutes to seven, before the fourteen hundred guests had gone to their tables, while everyone was still milling around drinking and talking. Taken to the reception room reserved for guests of honor, which as usual was filled with over a hundred people, most of whom weren't supposed to be there, Boone, after drinking a cocktail and undergoing a quantity of greetings and introductions, had asked for a private spot where he could look over his speech, and had been taken to a small room just off the stage. His wife, who had come with him to the dinner, had stayed in the reception room. His niece, Nina Boone, had gone along to the private spot to help with the speech if required, but he had almost immediately sent her back to the reception room to get herself another cocktail and she had remained there.

Shortly after Boone and his niece had departed for the murder room, as the papers called it, Phoebe Gunther had showed up. Miss Gunther was Boone's confidential secretary, and she had with her two can openers, two monkey wrenches, two shirts (men's), two fountain pens, and a baby carriage. These were to be used as exhibits by Boone for illustrating points in his speech, and Miss Gunther wanted to get them to him at once, so she was escorted to the murder room, the escort, a member of the NIA, wheeling the baby carriage, which contained the other items, to the astonished amusement of the multitude as they passed through. Miss Gunther remained with Boone only a couple of minutes, delivering the exhibits, and then returned to the reception room for a cocktail. She reported that Boone had said he wanted to be alone.

At seven-thirty everybody in the reception room was herded out to the ballroom, to find their places on the dais and at the tables, where the fourteen hundred were settling down and the waiters were ready to hurl themselves into the fray. About seven forty-five Mr. Alger Kates arrived. He was from the Research Department of the BPR, and he had some last-minute statistics which were to be used in Boone's speech. He came to the dais looking for Boone, and Mr. Frank Thomas Erskine, the President of NIA, had told a waiter to show him where Boone was. The waiter had led him through the door to backstage and pointed to the door of the murder room.

Alger Kates had discovered the body. It was on the floor, the head battered with one of the monkey wrenches, which was lying near by. The implication of what Kates did next had been hinted at in some newspapers, and openly stated in others: namely, that no BPR man would trust any NIA man in connection with anything whatever, including murder. Anyhow, instead of returning to the ballroom and the dais to impart the news, Kates had looked around backstage until he found a phone, called the hotel manager, and told him to come at once and bring all the policemen he could find.

By Thursday evening, forty-eight hours after the event, something like a thousand other details had been accumulated, as for instance that nothing but smudges were found on the handle of the monkey wrench, no identifiable prints, and so forth and so forth, but that was the main picture as it had been painted when I was typing my report.

7.

Friday we got the bite. Since Wolfe spends every morning from nine to eleven up in the plant rooms, I was in the office alone when the call came. The call took the regular routine in this Land of the Secretary.

"Miss Harding calling Mr. Wolfe. Put Mr. Wolfe on, please."

If I put it all down it would take half a page to get me, not Mr. Wolfe, just me, connected with Miss Harding. Anyhow I made it, and got the idea across that Wolfe was engaged with orchids and I would have to do. She wanted to know how soon Wolfe could get up there to see Mr. Erskine, and I explained that he seldom left the house for any purpose whatever, and never merely on business.

"I know that!" she snapped. She must have missed another night's sleep. "But this is *Mr. Erskine!*"

I knew we had him now, so I snooted her. "To you," I agreed, "he is all of that. To Mr. Wolfe he is nothing but a pest. Mr. Wolfe hates to work, even at home."

Instructed to hold the wire, I did so, for about ten minutes. Finally her voice came again:

"Mr. Goodwin?"

"Still here. Older and wiser, but still here."

"Mr. Erskine will be at Mr. Wolfe's office at four-thirty this afternoon."

I was getting exasperated. "Listen, Public Relations," I demanded, "why don't you simplify it by connecting me with this Erskine? If he comes at four-thirty he'll wait an hour and a half. Mr. Wolfe's hours with orchids are from nine to eleven in the morning and from four to six in the afternoon, and nothing short of murder—I mean nothing—has ever changed it or ever will."

"That's ridiculous!"

"Sure it is. So is this ring-around-the-rosy method for a man communicating with another man, but I stand for it."

"Hold the wire."

I never got connected with Erskine, that was too much to expect, but in spite of everything we finally completed an arrrangement, fighting our way through the obstacles, so that when Wolfe come downstairs at eleven o'clock I was able to announce to him:

"Mr. Frank Thomas Erskine, President of the National Industrial Association, with outriders, will be here at ten minutes past three."

"Satisfactory, Archie," he muttered.

Frankly, I wish I could make my heart quit doing an extra thump when Wolfe says satisfactory, Archie. It's childish.

3.

WHEN the doorbell rang that afternoon right on the dot at three-ten and I left my chair to answer it, I remarked to Wolfe:

"These people are apt to be the kind that you often walk out on or, even worse, tell me to eject. It may be necessary to control yourself. Remember the payroll. There is much at stake. Remember Fritz, Theodore, Charley, and me."

He didn't even grunt.

The catch was above expectations, for in the delegation of four we got not one Erskine but two. Father and son. Father was maybe sixty and struck me as not imposing. He was tall and bony and narrow, wearing a dark blue ready-made that didn't fit, and didn't have false teeth but talked as if he had. He handled the introductions, first himself and then the others. Son was named Edward Frank and addressed as Ed. The other two, certified as members of the NIA Executive Committee, were Mr. Breslow and Mr. Winterhoff. Breslow looked as if he had been born flushed with anger and would die, when the time came, in character. If it had not been beneath the dignity of a member of the NIA Executive Committee, Winderhoff could have snagged a fee posing as a Man of Distinction for a whisky ad. He even had the little gray mustache.

As for Son, not yet Ed to me, who was about my age, I reserved judgment because he apparently had a hangover and that is no time to file a man away. Unquestionably he had a headache. His suit had cost at least three times as much as Father's.

When I had got them distributed on chairs, with Father on the red leather number near the end of Wolfe's desk, at his elbow a small table just the right size for resting a checkbook on while writing in it, Father spoke:

"This may be time wasted for us, Mr. Wolfe. It seemed

impossible to get any satisfactory information on the telephone. Have you been engaged by anyone to investigate this matter?"

Wolfe lifted a brow a sixteenth of an inch. "What matter, Mr. Erskine?"

"Uh—this—the death of Cheney Boone."

Wolfe considered. "Let me put it this way. I have agreed to nothing and accepted no fee. I am committed to no interest."

"In a case of murder," Breslow sputtered angrily, "there is only one interest, the interest of justice."

"Oh, for God's sake," son Ed growled.

Father's eyes moved. "If necessary," he said emphatically, "the rest of you can leave and I'll do this alone." He returned to Wolfe. "What opinion have you formed about it?"

"Opinions, from experts, cost money."

"We'll pay you for it."

"A reasonable amount," Winterhoff put in. His voice was heavy and flat. He couldn't have been cast as a Man of Distinction with a sound-track.

"It wouldn't be worth even that," Wolfe said, "unless it were expert, and it wouldn't be expert unless I did some work. I haven't decided whether I shall go that far. I don't like to work."

"Who has consulted you?" Father wanted to know.

"Now, sir, really." Wolfe wiggled a finger at him. "It is indiscreet of you to ask, and I would be a blatherskite to answer. Did you come here with the notion of hiring me?"

"Well—" Erskine hesitated. "That has been discussed as a possibility."

"For you gentlemen as individuals, or on behalf of the National Industrial Association?"

"It was discussed as an Association matter."

Wolfe shook his head. "I would advise strongly against it. You might be wasting your money."

"Why? Aren't you a good investigator?"

"I am the best. But the situation is obvious. What you are concerned about is the reputation and standing of your Association. In the public mind the trial has already been held and the verdict rendered. Everyone knows that your Association was bitterly hostile to the Bureau of Price Regulation, to Mr. Boone, and to his policies. Nine people out of ten are confident that they know who murdered Mr. Boone. It was the National Industrial Association." Wolfe's eyes came to me. "Archie. What was it the man at the bank said?"

"Oh, just that gag that's going around. That NIA stands for Not Innocent Atall."

"But that's preposterous!"

"Certainly," Wolfe agreed, "but there it is. The NIA has been convicted and sentence has been pronounced. The only possible way of getting that verdict reversed would be to find the murderer and convict him. Even if it turned out that the murderer was a member of the NIA, the result would be the same; the interest and the odium would be transferred to the individual, if not altogether, at least to a great extent, and nothing else would transfer any of it."

They looked at one another. Winterhoff nodded gloomily and Breslow kept his lips compressed so as not to explode. Ed Erskine glared at Wolfe as if that was where his headache had come from.

"You say," Father told Wolfe, "that the public has convicted the NIA. But so have the police. So has the FBI. They are acting exactly like the Gestapo. The members of such an old and respectable organization as the NIA might be supposed to have some rights and privileges. Do you know what the police are doing? In addition to everything else, do you know that they are actually communicating with the police in every city in the United States? Asking them to get a signed statement from local citizens who were in New York at that dinner and have returned home?"

"Indeed," Wolfe said politely. "But I imagine the local police will furnish paper and ink."

"What?" Father stared at him.

"What the hell has that got to do with it?" Son wanted to know.

Wolfe skipped it and observed, "The deuce of it is that the probability that the police will catch the murderer seems somewhat thin. Not having studied the case thoroughly, I can't qualify as an expert on it, but I must say it looks doubtful. Three days and nights have passed. That's why I advise against your hiring me. I admit it would be worth almost any amount to your Association to have the murderer exposed, even it he proved to be one of you four gentlemen, but I would tackle the job, if at all, only with the greatest reluctance. I'm sorry you had your trip down here for nothing.—Archie?"

The implication being that I should show them what good manners we had by taking them to the front door, I stood up. They didn't. Instead they exchanged glances.

Winterhoff said to Erskine, "I would go ahead, Frank."

Breslow demanded, "What else can we do?"

Ed growled, "Oh, God, I wish he was alive again. That was better than this."

I sat down.

Erskine said, "We are businessmen, Mr. Wolfe. We understand that you can't guarantee anything. But if we persuade you to undertake this matter, exactly what would you engage to do?"

It took them nearly ten minutes to persuade him, and they all looked relieved, even Ed, when he finally gave in. It was more or less understood that the clinching argument was Breslow's, that they must not let justice down. Unfortunately, since the NIA had a voucher system, the check-writing table did not get used. As a substitute I typed a letter, dictated by Wolfe, and Erskine signed it. The retainer was to be ten thousand dollars, and the ultimate charge, including expenses, was left open. They certainly were on the ropes.

"Now," Erskine said, handing me back my fountain pen, "I suppose we had better tell you all we know about it."

Wolfe shook his head. "Not right now. I have to get my mind adjusted to this confounded mess. It would be better for you to return this evening, say at nine o'clock."

They all protested. Winterhoff said he had an appointment he couldn't break.

"As you please, sir. If it is more important than this. We must get to work without delay." Wolfe turned to me: "Archie, your notebook. A telegram. 'You are invited to join in a discussion of the Boone murder at the office of Nero Wolfe at nine o'clock this evening Friday March twenty-ninth.' Sign it with my name. Send it at once to Mr. Cramer, Mr. Spero, Mr. Kates, Miss Gunther, Mrs. Boone, Miss Nina Boone, Mr. Rohde, and perhaps to others, we'll see later.—Will you gentlemen be here?"

"My God," Ed grumbled, "with that mob, why don't you hold it in the Grand Ballroom at the Waldorf?"

"It seems to me," Erskine said in a grieved tone, "that this is a mistake. The first principle—"

"I," Wolfe said, in a tone used by NIA men only to people whose names were never on the letterhead, "am handling the investigation."

I started banging the typewriter, and since the telegrams were urgent, and since Wolfe took long walks only in emergencies, Fritz was sent for to escort them to the door. All I was typing was the text of the telegram and a list of the names and addresses, because the phone was the quickest way to send them. Some of the addresses were a problem. Wolfe was leaning back in his chair with his eyes closed, not to be bothered about trivialities, so I called Lon Cohen on the city desk at the *Gazette* and got the addresses from him. He knew everything. They had come up from Washington for the big speech that was never delivered and had not gone back. Mrs. Boone and the niece were at the Waldorf,

Alger Kates was staying with friends on Eleventh Street, and Phoebe Gunther, who had been Boone's confidential secretary, had a room-and-bath on East Fifty-fifth Street.

When I had that job done I asked Wolfe who else he wanted to invite. He said no one. I stood up and stretched, and looked at him.

"I presume," I observed, "that the rest is merely routine collection of evidence. Ed Erskine has calluses on his hands. Will that help?"

"Confound it." He sighed clear down. "I was going to finish that book this evening. Now this infernal mish-mash."

He heaved the bulk forward and rang for beer.

I, standing at the cabinet filing the germination records that Theodore had brought down from the plant rooms, was compelled to admit that he had earned my admiration. Not for his conception of the idea of digging up a paying customer; that was merely following precedent in times of drought. Not for the method he had adopted for the digging; I could have thought that up myself. Not for the execution, his handling of the NIA delegation; that was an obvious variation of the old hard-to-get finesse. Not for the gall of those telegrams; admiring Wolfe's gall would be like admiring ice at the North Pole or green leaves in a tropical jungle. No. What I admired was his common sense. He wanted to get a look at those people. What do you do when you want to get a look at a man? You get your hat and go where he is. But what if the idea of getting your hat and going outdoors is abhorrent to you? You ask the man to come where you are. What makes you think he'll come? That was where the common sense entered. Take Inspector Cramer. Why would he, the head of the Homicide Squad, come? Because he didn't know how long Wolfe had been on the case or how deep he was in it, and therefore he couldn't afford to stay away.

At four sharp Wolfe had downed the last of his beer and taken the elevator up to the plant rooms. I finished the filing and gathered up miscellaneous loose ends around the office, expecting to be otherwise engaged for at least a day or two, and then settled down at my desk with a stack of newspaper clippings to make sure I hadn't missed anything important in my typed summary of the Boone situation. I was deep in that when the doorbell rang, and I went to the front and opened up, and found confronting me a vacuum cleaner salesman. Or anyhow he should have been. He had that bright, friendly, uninhibited look. But some of the details didn't fit, as for example his clothes, which were the kind I would begin buying when my rich uncle died.

"Hello!" he said cheerfully. "I'll bet you're Archie Goodwin. You came to see Miss Harding yesterday. She told me about you. Aren't you Archie Goodwin?"

"Yep," I said. It was the easiest way out. If I had said no or tried to evade he would have cornered me sooner or later.

"I thought so." He was gratified. "May I come in? I'd like to see Mr. Wolfe. I'm Don O'Neill, but of course that doesn't mean anything to you. I'm president of O'Neill and Warder, Incorporated, and a member of that godforsaken conglomeration of antiques, the NIA. I was Chairman of the Dinner Committee for that affair we had at the Waldorf the other evening. I guess I'll never live that one down. Chairman of a Dinner Committee, and let the main speaker get murdered!"

Of course my reaction was that I had got along fairly well for something like thirty years without knowing Don O'Neill and saw no reason for a change in policy, but my personal feelings could not be permitted to dominate. So I let him in and steered him to the office and into a chair before I even explained that he would have to wait half an hour because Wolfe was engaged. For a brief moment he seemed irritated, but he realized instantly that that was no way to sell vacuum cleaners and said sure, that was all right, he didn't mind waiting.

He was delighted with the office and got up and went around looking. Books—what a selection! The big globe was marvelous, just what he had always wanted and never took the trouble to get one, now he would . . .

Wolfe entered, saw him, and gave me a dirty look. It was true that I was supposed to inform him in advance of any waiting caller and never let him come in cold like that, but it was ten to one that if I had told him about O'Neill he would have refused to see him and had me invite him for the nine o'clock party, and I saw no necessity for another three-hour rest for Wolfe's brains. He was so sore that he pretended he didn't believe in shaking hands, acknowledged the introduction with a nod that wouldn't have spilled a drop if he had had a jar of water on his head, sat down and regarded the visitor unsympathetically, and asked curtly:

"Well, sir?"

O'Neill wasn't at all taken aback. He said, "I was admiring your office."

"Thank you. But I assume that wasn't what you came for."

"Oh, no. Being the Chairman of that Dinner Committee, I'm in the middle of this thing whether I like it or not—this business of Boone's murder. I wouldn't say I'm involved, that's too strong a word—make it concerned. I'm certainly concerned."

"Has anyone suggested that you are involved?"

"Suggested?" O'Neill looked surprised. "That's putting it mildly. The police are taking the position that everyone connected with the NIA is involved. That's why I claim that the line the Executive Committee is taking is sentimental and unrealistic. Don't get me wrong, Mr. Wolfe." He took time out for a friendly glance at me, to include me in the Society of United Citizens for Not Getting Don O'Neill Wrong. "I am one of the most progressive members of the NIA. I was a Willkie man. But this idea of co-operating with the police the way they're acting, and even spending our own money to investigate, that's unrealistic. We ought to say to the police, all right, there's been a murder, and as good citizens we hope you catch the guilty man, but we had nothing to do with it and it's none of our business."

"And tell them to quit bothering you."

"That's right. That's exactly right." O'Neill was pleased to find a kindred spirit. "I was at the office when they came back an hour ago with the news that they had engaged you to investigate. I want to make it plain that I am not doing anything underhanded. I don't work that way. We had another argument, and I told them I was coming to see you."

"Admirable." Wolfe's eyes were open, which meant that he was bored and was getting nothing out of it. Either that, or he was refusing to turn on the brain until nine o'clock. "For the purpose of persuading me to call it off?"

"Oh, no. I saw that was hopeless. You wouldn't do that. Would you?"

"I'm afraid not without some excellent reason. As Mr. Breslow put it, the interest of justice is paramount. That was his position. Mine is that I need the money. Then what did you come for?"

O'Neill grinned at me, as if to say, your boss is really a card, isn't he? He shifted the grin intact to Wolfe. "I'm glad to see you stick to the point. With me you need to, the way I go floundering around. What brought me down here, frankly, was a sense of my responsibility as Chairman of the Dinner Committee. I've seen a copy of the letter Frank Erskine gave you, but I didn't hear the conversation you had, and ten thousand dollars as a retainer on a straight inquiry job is away above the clouds. I hire detectives in my business, things like labor relations and so on, and I know what detectives get, so naturally the question occurs to me, is it really a straight inquiry job? I asked Erskine point-blank, have you hired Wolfe to protect the NIA members by—uh—

getting attention shifted to other directions, and he said no. But I know Frank Erskine, and I wasn't satisfied, and I told him so. The trouble with me is I've got a conscience and a sense of responsibility. So I came to ask you."

Wolfe's lips twitched, but whether with amusement or fierce indignation I couldn't tell. The way he takes an insult never depends on the insult but on how he happens to be feeling. At the peak of one of his lazy spells he wouldn't have exerted himself to bat an eyelash even if someone accused him of specializing in divorce evidence.

His lips twitched. "I also say no, Mr. O'Neill. But I'm afraid that won't help you much. What if Mr. Erskine and I are both lying? I don't see what you can do about it, short of going to the police and charging us with obstructing justice, but then you don't like the police either. You're really in a pickle. We have invited some people to meet here this evening at nine o'clock and talk it over. Why don't you come and keep an eye on us?"

"Oh, I'm coming. I told Erskine and the others I'm coming."

"Good. Then we won't keep you now.—Archie?"

It wasn't as simple as that. O'Neill was by no means ready to go, on account of his sense of responsibility. But we finally got him out without resorting to physical violence. After wrangling him to the stoop, I returned to the office and asked Wolfe:

"Exactly what did he really come here for? Of course he killed Boone, I understand that, but why did he waste his time and mine—"

"You let him in," Wolfe said icily. "You did not notify me. You seem to forget—"

"Oh, well," I broke in cheerfully, "it all helps in studying human nature. I helped get him out, didn't I? Now we have work to do, getting ready for the party. How many will there be, around twelve not counting us?"

I got busy on the chair problem. There were six there in the office, and the divan would hold four comfortably, except that in a murder case three days old you don't often find four people connected with it who are still in a frame of mind to sit together on the same piece of furniture. It would be better to have plenty of chairs, so I brought five more in from the front room, the one facing on the street, and scattered them around, not in rows, which would have been too stiff, but sort of staggered and informal. Big as the room was, it made it look pretty crowded. I backed against the wall and surveyed it with a frown.

"What it needs," I remarked, "is a woman's touch."

"Bah," Wolfe growled.

9.

AT a quarter past ten Wolfe was leaning back in his chair with his eyes half closed, taking them in. They had been at it for over an hour.

There were thirteen of them. Thanks to my foresight with the seating arrangements, there had been no infighting. The NIA contingent was at the side of the room farthest from my desk, the side toward the hall door, with Erskine in the red leather chair. There were six of them: the four who had formed the afternoon delegation, including Winterhoff, who had had an appointment he couldn't break, Hattie Harding, and Don O'Neill.

On my side of the room were the BPR's, four in number: Mrs. Boone the widow, Nina the niece, Alger Kates, and a gate-crasher named Solomon Dexter. Dexter was around fifty, under rather than over, looked like a cross between a statesman and a lumberjack, and was the ex-Deputy Director, now for twenty-four hours Acting Director, of the Bureau of Price Regulation. He had come, he told Wolfe, ex officio.

In between the two hostile armies were the neutrals or referees: Spero of the FBI, and Inspector Cramer and Sergeant Purley Stebbins. I had explained to Cramer that I was aware that he rated the red leather chair, but that he was needed in the middle. By a quarter past ten he was about as mad as I had ever seen him, because he had long ago caught on that Wolfe was starting from scratch and had arranged the gathering for the purpose of taking in, not giving out.

There had been one puny attempt to disrupt my seating plans. Mrs. Boone and the niece had come early, before nine, and since there is nothing wrong with my eyesight I had without the slightest hesitation put the niece in the chair—one of the yellow ones from the front room—nearest to mine. When Ed Erskine arrived, alone, a little later, I assigned him to a seat on the NIA side, only to discover, after attending to a couple of other customers, that he had bounced across and was in my chair talking to the niece. I went over and told him:

"This side is for the Capulets. Would you mind sitting where I put you?"

He twisted his neck and lifted his chin to get me, and his focusing was not good. It was obvious that he had been applying the theory of acquired immunity to his hangover. I want to be fair, he was not pie-eyed, but neither was he in danger of desiccating.

He asked me, "Huh? Why?"

"Besides," I said, "this is my chair and I work here. Let's not make an issue of it."

He shrugged it off and moved. I addressed Nina Boone courteously:

"You run into all sorts of strangers in a detective's office."

"I suppose you do," she said. Not a deep remark, nothing specially penetrating about it, but I smiled at her to show I appreciated her taking the trouble to make it when under a strain. She had dark hair and eyes, and was keeping her chin firm.

From the moment, right at the beginning, that Wolfe had announced that he had been retained by the NIA, the BPR's had been suspicious and antagonistic. Of course everyone who reads a newspaper or listens to the radio, which includes me, knew that the NIA hated Cheney Boone and all he stood for, and had done everything possible to get him tossed to the wolves, and also knew that the BPR would gladly have seen the atom bomb tested by bunching the NIA crowd on an island and dropping one on them, but I hadn't realized how it sizzled until that evening in Wolfe's office. Of course there were two fresh elements in it then: the fact that Cheney Boone had been murdered, at an NIA dinner of all places, and the prospect that some person or persons either would or wouldn't get arrested, tried, convicted, and electrocuted.

By a quarter past ten a good many points, both trivial and important, had been touched on. On opportunity, the BPR position was that everyone in the reception room, and probably many others, had known that Boone was in the room near the stage, the murder room, while the NIA claimed that not more than four or five people, besides the BPR's who were there, knew it. The truth was that there was no way of finding out who had known and who hadn't.

Neither hotel employees nor anyone else had heard any noise from the murder room, or seen anybody enter or leave it other than those whose presence there was known and acknowledged.

No one was eliminated on account of age, size, or sex. While a young male athlete can swing a monkey wrench harder and faster than an old female bridge player, either could have struck the blows that killed Boone. There had been no sign of a struggle. Any one of the blows, from behind, could have stunned him or killed him. G. G. Spero of the FBI joined in the discussion of this point, and replied to a crack from Erskine by stating that it was not a function of the FBI to investigate local murders, but that since Boone had been killed while performing his duty as a government official, the Department of Justice had a legitimate interest in the matter and was acting on a request for co-operation from the New York police.

One interesting development was that it was hard to see how Boone had got killed unless he did it himself, because everybody had alibis. Meaning by everybody not merely those present in Wolfe's office—there being no special reason to suppose that the murderer was there with us—but all of the fourteen or fifteen hundred at the dinner. The time involved was about half an hour, between seven-fifteen, when Phoebe Gunther left the baby carriage and its contents, including the monkey wrenches, with Boone in the room, and around seven forty-five, when Alger Kates discovered the body. The police had gone to town on that, and everybody had been with somebody else, especially those in the reception room. But the hitch was that all the alibis were either mutual NIA's or mutual BPR's. Strange to say, no NIA could alibi a BPR, or vice versa. Even Mrs. Boone, the widow, for instance —no NIA was quite positive that she had not left the reception room during that period or that she had gone straight from there to the dais in the ballroom. The BPR's were equally unpositive about Frank Thomas Erskine, the NIA president.

There was no evidence that the purpose had been to keep Boone from delivering that particular speech. The speech had been typical Boone, pulling no punches, but had exposed or threatened no particular individual, neither in the advance text distributed to the press nor in the last-minute changes and additions. Nothing in it pointed to a murderer.

The first brand-new ingredient for me, of which nothing had been reported in the papers, was introduced by accident by Mrs. Boone. The only person invited to our party who hadn't come was Phoebe Gunther, Boone's confidential secretary. Her name had of course been mentioned several times during the first hour or so, but it was Mrs. Boone who put the spotlight on it. I had the notion that she did it deliberately. She had not up to that moment got any of my major attention. She was mature and filled-out, though not actually fat and by no means run to seed, and she had been short-changed as to nose.

Wolfe had doubled back to the question of Cheney Boone's

arrival at the Waldorf, and Cramer, who was by then in a frame of mind to get it over with and disperse, had said sarcastically, "I'll send you a copy of my notes. Meanwhile Goodwin can take this down. Five of them—Boone and his wife, Nina Boone, Phoebe Gunther, and Alger Kates—were to take the one o'clock train from Washington to New York, but Boone got caught in an emergency conference and couldn't make it. The other four came on the train, and when they reached New York Mrs. Boone went to the Waldorf, where rooms had been engaged, and the other three went to the BPR New York office. Boone came on a plane that landed at LaGuardia Field at six-five, went to the hotel and up to the room where his wife was. By that time the niece was there too, and the three of them went together down to the ballroom floor. They went straight to the reception room. Boone had no hat or coat to check, and he hung onto a little leather case he had with him."

"That was the case," Mrs. Boone put in, "that Miss Gunther *says* she forgot about and left on a window sill."

I looked at the widow reproachfully. That was the first sign of a split in the BPR ranks, and it sounded ominous, with the nasty emphasis she put on *says*. To make it worse, Hattie Harding of the NIA immediately picked it up:

"And Miss Gunther is absolutely wrong, because four different people saw that case in her hand as she left the reception room!"

Solomon Dexter snorted. "It's amazing what—"

"Please, sir." Wolfe wiggled a finger at him. "What was this case? A brief case? A vanity case?"

"No." Cramer was helping out again. "It was a little leather case like a doctor's, and it contained cylinders from a dictating machine. Miss Gunther has described it to me. When she took that baby carriage and other stuff to him Tuesday evening, to the room where he was killed, he told her the conference in Washington had ended earlier than he expected, and he had gone to his office and spent an hour dictating before he took the plane to New York. He had the cylinders with him in that case for her to transcribe. She took it to the reception room when she went back there for a cocktail, and left it there on a window sill. That's the last of it."

"So she says," Mrs. Boone repeated.

Dexter glared at her. "Nonsense!"

"Did *you,*" Hattie Harding demanded, "see the case in her hand when she left the reception room?"

All eyes went to the widow. She moved hers and got the picture. One word would be enough. She was either a traitor or she wasn't. Confronted with that alternative, it didn't take her long to decide. She met Hattie Harding's gaze and said distinctly:

"No."

Everybody breathed. Wolfe asked Cramer:

"What was on the cylinders, letters? What?"

"Miss Gunther doesn't know. Boone didn't tell her. No one in Washington knows."

"The conference that ended earlier than Boone expected, what was it about?"

Cramer shook his head.

"Who was it with?"

Cramer shook his head again. G. G. Spero offered, "We've been working on that in Washington. We can't trace any conference. We don't know where Boone was for about two hours, from one to three. The best lead is that the head NIA man in Washington had been wanting to see him, to discuss his speech, but he denies—"

Breslow exploded. "By God," he blurted, "there it is! It's always an NIA man! That's damned silly, Spero, and don't forget where FBI salaries come from! They come from taxpayers!"

From that point on the mud was flying more or less constantly. It wasn't on account of any encouragement from Wolfe. He told Breslow:

"The constant reference to your Association is unfortunate from your standpoint, sir, but it can't be helped. A murder investigation invariably centers on people with motives. You heard Mr. Cramer, early in this discussion, say that a thorough inquiry has disclosed no evidence of personal enemies. But you cannot deny that Mr. Boone had many enemies, earned by his activities as a government official, and that a large number of them were members of the NIA."

Winterhoff asked, "A question, Mr. Wolfe, is it always an enemy who kills a man?"

"Answer it yourself," Wolfe told him. "Obviously that's what you asked it for."

"Well, it certainly isn't always an enemy," Winterhoff declared. "For an illustration, you couldn't say that Mr. Dexter here was Boone's enemy, quite the contrary, they were friends. But if Mr. Dexter had been filled with ambition to become the Director of the Bureau of Price Regulation—and that's what he is at this moment—he might conceivably have taken steps to make the office vacant. Incidentally, he would also have placed under grave suspicion the members of an organization he mortally hates—which also has happened."

Solomon Dexter was smiling at him, not a loving smile. "Are you preferring a charge, Mr. Winterhoff?"

"Not at all." The other met his gaze. "As I said, merely an illustration."

"Because I could mention one little difficulty. I was in Washington until eleven o'clock Tuesday evening. You'll have to get around that somehow."

"Nevertheless," Frank Thomas Erskine said firmly and judicially, "Mr. Winterhoff has made an obvious point."

"One of several," Breslow asserted. "There are others. We all know what they are, so why not out with them? The talk about Boone and his secretary, Phoebe Gunther, has been going on for months, and whether Mrs. Boone was going to get a divorce or not. And lately a reason, a mighty good reason from Phoebe Gunther's standpoint, why Boone had to have a divorce no matter how his wife felt about it. What about it, Inspector, when you're dealing with a murder don't you think it's legitimate to take an interest in things like that?"

Alger Kates stood up and announced in a trembling voice: "I want to protest that this is utterly despicable and beyond the bounds of common decency!"

His face was white and he stayed on his feet. I had not supposed he had it in him. He was the BPR research man who had taken some up-to-the-minute statistics to the Waldorf to be used in Boone's speech and had discovered the body. If my attention had been directed to him on the subway and I had been asked to guess what he did for a living, I would have said, "Research man." He was that to a T, in size, complexion, age, and chest measurement. But the way he rose to protest—apparently he led the BPR, as there represented, in spunk. I grinned at him.

From the reaction he got you might have thought that what the NIA hated and feared most about the BPR was its research. They all howled at him. I caught the gist of only two of their remarks, one from Breslow to the effect that he had only said what everyone was saying, and the wind-up from Don O'Neill, in the accents of The Boss:

"You can keep out of this, Kates! Sit down and shut up!"

That seemed to me to be overdoing it a little, since he wasn't paying Kates's wages; and then Erskine, twisting around in the red leather chair to face the research man, told him cuttingly:

"Since you didn't regard the President of the NIA as a fit person to bring the news to, you are hardly acceptable as a judge of common decency."

So, I thought, that's why they're jumping on him, because he told the hotel manager instead of them. He should have had more sense than to hurt their feelings like that. Erskine wasn't through with him, but was going on:

"Surely, Mr. Kates, you are aware that personal emotions, such as jealousy, revenge, or frustration, often result in violence, and therefore they are proper matters of inquiry when a murder has been committed. It would be proper to ask you, for example, whether it is true that you wanted to marry Boone's niece, and you were aware that Boone opposed it and intended to prevent—"

"Why, you big liar!" Nina Boone cried.

"Whether it is proper or not," Kates said in a high thin voice that was still trembling, "it certainly is not proper for you to ask me anything whatever. If I were asked that by the police, I would reply that part of it is true and part of it isn't. There are at least two hundred men in the BPR organization who wanted, and it is a reasonable assumption that they still want, to marry Mr. Boone's niece. I was not under the impression that Mr. Boone was having anything to say about it one way or another, and, knowing Miss Boone as I do, not intimately but fairly well, I doubt it." Kates moved not his eyes, but his head, to change his target. "I would like to ask Mr. Wolfe, who has admitted that he is in the pay of the NIA, if we were invited here for a typical NIA inquisition."

"And I," Solomon Dexter put in, his voice sounding like a train in a tunnel in contrast to Kates's, "would like to inform you, Mr. Wolfe, that you are by no means the only detective in the employ of the NIA. For nearly a year executives and other BPR personnel have been followed by detectives, and their whole lives have been thoroughly explored in an effort to get something on them. I don't know whether you have taken part in those operations—"

More bedlam from the NIA, taking the form chiefly, as near as I could get it, of indignant denials. At that point, if it hadn't been for my seating arrangements, the two armies would probably have made contact. Wolfe was looking exasperated, but making no effort to stop it, possibly aware that it would take more energy than he wished to spend. What quieted them was Inspector Cramer getting to his feet and showing a palm, officially.

"*I* would like," he barked, "before going, to say three things. First, Mr. Dexter, I can assure you that Wolfe has not helped to tail your personnel or explore their lives, because there's not enough money in that kind of work. Second, Mr. Erskine and you other gentlemen, the police are aware that jealousy and things like that are often behind a murder, and we are not apt to forget it. Third, Mr. Kates, I have known Wolfe for twenty years, and I can tell you why you were invited here this evening. We were invited because he wanted to learn all he could as quick as he could, without leaving his chair and without Goodwin's buying gas and wearing out his tires. I don't know about the rest of you, but I was a sucker to come."

He turned. "Come on, Sergeant. You coming, Spero?"

Of course that ended it. The BPR didn't want any more anyhow, and though the NIA, or part of it, showed an inclination to stay and make suggestions, Wolfe used his veto power on that. With everyone out of their chairs, Ed Erskine crossed the lines again and tried another approach on Nina, but it appeared, from where I stood, that she disposed of that without even opening her mouth. I did much better, in spite of my being associated with Wolfe, who was in the pay of the NIA. When I told her that it was impossible to get a taxi in that part of town and offered to drive her and her aunt to their hotel, she said:

"Mr. Dexter is taking us."

A frank, friendly statement, and I appreciated it.

But after they had all gone and Wolfe and I were alone in the office, it appeared that I wouldn't have been able to go through with it even if she had accepted. I remarked to Wolfe:

"Too bad Cramer bolixed it up like that. If we had been able to keep them here a while, say two weeks, we might have got started somewhere. Too bad."

"It was not too bad," he said testily.

"Oh." I gestured, and sat down. "Okay, then it was a screaming success. Of all our guests, which do you think was the most interesting?"

To my surprise, he answered, "The most interesting was Miss Gunther."

"Yeah? Because?"

"Because she didn't come. You have her address."

"Sure. I sent the telegram—"

"Go and bring her here."

I stared at him, looked at my wrist, and stared at him again. "It is now twenty minutes past eleven."

He nodded. "The streets are less dangerous at night, with the reduced traffic."

"I won't argue." I stood up. "You are in the pay of the NIA, and I am in the pay of you. So it goes."

10.

I TOOK an assortment of keys along, to simplify things in case 611 East Fifty-fifth Street proved to be an old-fashioned walk-up with a locked entrance door, but instead of that it was one of the twelve-story beehives with an awning and hired men. I stepped down the broad hall to the elevator, went in, and said casually:

"Gunther."

Without even glancing at me, the pilot finished a yawn and called out, "Hey, Sam! For Gunther!"

The doorman, whom I had by-passed, appeared and looked in at me. "I'll phone up," he said, "but it's a waste of time. What's your name and what paper are you from?"

Ordinarily I like to save butter, but under the circumstances, with no ceiling on expenses, I saw no reason why he shouldn't be in the pay of the NIA too. So I left the elevator and walked down the hall with him, and when we got to the switchboard I spread a ten-dollar bill thereon, saying:

"I'm not on a paper. I sell sea shells."

He shook his head and started manipulations at the board. I put a hand on his arm and told him, "You didn't let me finish. That was papa. Here's mamma." I deployed another ten. "But I warn you they have no children."

He only shook his head again and flipped a lever. I was shocked speechless. I have had a lot to do with doormen, and I am certainly able to spot one too honest to accept twenty bucks for practically nothing, and that was not it. His principles didn't even approach as high a standard as that, and he was being pure from some other motive. I emerged from the shock when I heard him telling the receiver:

"He says he sells sea shells."

"The name," I said, "is Archie Goodwin, and I was sent by Mr. Nero Wolfe."

He repeated it to the receiver, and in a moment hung up and turned to me with a look of surprise. "She says go on up. Nine H." He accompanied me toward the elevator. "About papa and mamma, I've changed my mind, in case you still feel—"

"I was kidding you," I told him. "They really have got children. This is little Horace." I handed him two bits and went in and commanded the pilot, "Nine H."

It is not my custom to make personal remarks to young women during the first five minutes after meeting them, and if I violated it this time it was only because the remark popped out of me involuntarily. When I pushed the button and she opened the door and said good evening, and I agreed and removed my hat and stepped inside, the ceiling light right above her was shining on her hair, and what popped out was:

"Golden Bantam."

"Yes," she said, "that's what I dye it with."

I was already understanding, from the first ten seconds, what motive it was that the doorman was being pure from. Her pictures in the papers had been just nothing compared with this. After we had disposed of my hat and coat she preceded me into the room, and from the middle of it turned her head to say:

"You know Mr. Kates."

I thought it had popped out of her as my remark had popped out of me, but then I saw him, rising to his feet from a chair in a corner where the light was dim.

"Hello," I said.

"Good evening," he piped.

"Sit down." Phoebe Gunther straightened a corner of a rug with the toe of a little red slipper. "Mr. Kates came to tell me what happened at your party this evening. Will you have some Scotch? Rye? Bourbon? Gin? Cola?"

"No, thanks." I was getting my internal skull fixtures jerked back into place.

"Well." She sat on a couch against a nest of cushions. "Did you come to see what color my hair is or was there something else?"

"I'm sorry to bust in on you and Mr. Kates."

"That's all right. Isn't it, Al?"

"It is not all right," Alger Kates said, without hesitation, in his thin voice stretched tight but extremely distinct, "with me. It would be folly to trust him at all or to believe anything he says. As I told you, he is in the pay of the NIA."

"So you did." Miss Gunther was relaxing among the cushions. "But since we know enough not to trust him, all we have to do is to be a little smarter than he is in order to get more out of him than he gets out of us." She looked at me, and seemed to be smiling, but I had already discovered that her face was so versatile, especially her mouth, that it would be better not to jump to conclusions. She told me, possibly smiling, "I have a theory about Mr. Kates. He talks the way people talked before he was born, therefore he must read old-fashioned novels. I wouldn't suppose a research man would read novels at all. What would you suppose?"

"I don't discuss people who don't trust me," I said politely. "And I don't think you are."

"Are what?"

"Smarter than me. I admit you're prettier, but I doubt if you're smarter. I was spelling champion of Zanesville, Ohio, at the age of twelve."

"Spell snoop."

"That's just childish." I glared at her. "I don't imagine you're hinting that catching people who commit crimes is work to be ashamed of, since you're smart, so if what you have in mind is my coming here, why didn't you tell the doorman—"

I stopped short because she was possibly laughing at me. I quit glaring, but went on looking at her, which was a bad policy because that was what was interfering with my mental processes.

"Okay," I said curtly, "you got a poke in and made me blink. Round One for you. Round Two. Your Mr. Kates may be as loyal as What's-his-name, the boy that stood on the burning deck, but he's a sap. Nero Wolfe is tricky, that I admit, but the idea that he would cover a murderer because he happened to belong to something out of the alphabet that signed checks is plain loony. Look at the record and show me where he ever accepted a substitute, no matter who said it was just as good. Here's a free tip: if you think or know a BPR man did it, and don't want him caught, bounce me out immediately and keep as far away from Wolfe as you can get. If you think an NIA man did it and you'd like to help, put on some shoes and get your hat and coat and come to his office with me. As far as I'm concerned you don't need to bother about the hat." I looked at Kates. "If you did it yourself, with some motive not to be mentioned for the sake of common decency, you'd better come along and confess and get it over with."

"I told you!" Kates told her triumphantly. "See how he led up to that?"

"Don't be silly." Miss Gunther, annoyed, looked at him. "I'll explain it to you. Finding that I am smarter than he is, he decided to pick on you, and he certainly got documentation for his statement that you're a sap. In fact, you'd better be going. Leave him to me. I may see you at the office tomorrow."

Kates shook his head bravely and firmly. "No!" he insisted. "He'll go on that way! I'm not going to—"

He continued, but there's no more use my putting it down than there was his saying it, for the hostess had got up, crossed to a table, and picked up his hat and coat. It seemed to me that in some respects she must have been unsatisfactory as a confidential secretary. A man's secretary is always moving around, taking and bringing papers, ushering in callers and out again, sitting down and standing up, and if there is a constant temptation to watch how she moves it is hard to get any work done.

Kates lost the argument, of course. Within two minutes the door had closed behind him and Miss Gunther was back on the couch among the cushions. Meanwhile I had been doing my best to concentrate, so when she possibly smiled at me and told me to go ahead and teach her the multiplication table, I arose and asked if I might use her phone.

Her brows went up. "What am I supposed to do? Ask who you want to call?"

"No, just say yes."

"Yes. It's right over—"

"I see it, thanks."

It was on a little table against a wall, with a stool there, and I pulled out the stool and sat with my back to her and dialed. After only one buzz in my ear, because Wolfe hates to hear bells ring, I got a hello and spoke:

"Mr. Wolfe? Archie. I'm up here with Miss Gunther in her apartment, and I don't believe it's a good plan to bring her down there as you suggested. In the first place she's extremely smart, but that's not it. She's the one I've been dreaming about the past ten years, remember what I've told you? I don't mean she's beautiful, that's merely a matter of taste, I only mean she is exactly what I have had in mind. Therefore it will be much better to let me handle her. She began by making a monkey of me, but that was because I was suffering from shock. It may take a week or a month or even a year, because it is very difficult to keep your mind on your work under these circumstances, but you can count on me. You go on to bed and I'll get in touch with you in the morning."

I arose from the stool and turned to face the couch, but she wasn't there. She was, instead, over toward the door, in a dark blue coat with a fox collar, standing in front of a mirror, adjusting a dark blue contraption on her head.

She glanced at me. "All right, come on."

"Come on where?"

"Don't be demure." She turned from the mirror. "You worked hard trying to figure out a way of getting me down to Nero Wolfe's office, and you did a good job. I'll give you Round Two. Some day we'll play the rubber. Right now I'm taking on Nero Wolfe, so it will have to be postponed. I'm glad you don't think I'm beautiful. Nothing irritates a woman more than to be thought beautiful."

I had my coat on and she had the door open. The bag under her arm was the same dark blue material as the hat. On the way to the elevator I explained, "I didn't say I didn't think you were beautiful. I said—"

"I heard what you said. It stabbed me clear through. Even from a stranger who may also be my enemy, it hurt. I'm vain and that's that. Because it just happens that I can't see straight and I do think I'm beautiful."

"So do—" I began, but just in time I saw the corner of her mouth moving and bit it off. I am telling this straight. If anyone thinks I was muffing everything she sent my way I won't argue, but I would like to point out that I was right there with her, looking at her and listening to her, and the hell of it was that she *was* beautiful.

Driving down to Thirty-fifth Street, she kept the atmosphere as neighborly as if I had never been within ten miles of the NIA. Entering the house, we found the office uninhabited, so I left her there and went to find Wolfe. He was in the kitchen, deep in a conference with Fritz regarding the next day's culinary program, and I sat on a stool, thinking over the latest development, Gunther by name, until they were finished. Wolfe finally acknowledged my presence.

"Is she here?"

"Yep. She sure is. Straighten your tie and comb your hair."

11.

It was a quarter past two in the morning when Wolfe glanced at the wall clock, sighed, and said, "Very well, Miss Gunther, I am ready to fufill my part of the bargain. It was agreed that after you had answered my questions I would answer yours. Go ahead."

I hadn't been distracted much by gazing at beauty because, having been told to get it in the notebook verbatim, my eyes had been busy elsewhere. It was fifty-four pages. Wolfe had been in one of his looking-under-every-stone moods, and the stuff on some of the pages had no more to do with Boone's murder, from where I sat, than Washington crossing the Delaware.

Some of it might conceivably help. First and foremost, of course, was her own itinerary for last Tuesday. She knew nothing about the conference which had prevented Boone from leaving Washington on the train with the others, and admitted that that was surprising, since she was his confidential secretary and was supposed to know everything and usually did. Arriving in New York, she had gone with Alger Kates and Nina Boone to the BPR New York office, where Kates had gone into the statistical section, and she and Nina had helped department heads to collect props to be used as illustrations of points in the speech. There had been a large collection of all sorts of things, from toothpicks to typewriters, and it wasn't until after six o'clock that the final selection had been made: two can openers, two monkey wrenches, two shirts, two fountain pens, and a baby carriage; and the data on them assembled. One of the men had conveyed them to the street for her and found a taxi, and she had headed for the Waldorf, Nina having gone previously. A bellboy had helped her get the props to the ballroom floor and the reception room. There she learned that Boone had asked for privacy to go over his speech, and an NIA man, General Erskine, had taken her to the room, to be known before long as the murder room.

Wolfe asked, "*General* Erskine?"

"Yes," she said, "Ed Erskine, the son of the NIA President."

I snorted.

"He was a B.G.," she said. "One of the youngest generals in the Air Force."

"Do you know him well?"

"No, I had only seen him once or twice and had never met him. But naturally I hate him." At that moment there was no question about it; she was not smiling. "I hate everybody connected with the NIA."

"Naturally. Go ahead."

Ed Erskine had wheeled the baby carriage to the door of the room and left her there, and she had not stayed with Boone more than two or three minutes. The police had spent hours on those two or three minutes, since they were the last that anyone except the murderer had spent with Boone alive. Wolfe spent two pages of my notebook. Boone had been concentrated and tense, even more than usual, which was not remarkable under the circumstances. He had jerked the shirts and monkey wrenches out of the baby carriage and put them on the table, glanced at the data, reminded Miss Gunther that she was to follow a copy of the speech as he talked and take notes of any deviation he made from the text; and then had handed her the leather case and told her to get. She had returned to the reception room and had two cocktails, two quick ones because she felt she needed them, and then had joined the exodus to the ballroom and had found table number eight, the one near the dais reserved for BPR people. She was eating her fruit cocktail when she remembered about the leather case, and that she had left it on the window sill in the reception room. She said nothing about it because she didn't want to confess her carelessness, and just as she was starting to excuse herself to Mrs. Boone and leave the table, Frank Thomas Erskine, on the dais, had spoken into the microphone:

"Ladies and gentlemen, I regret the necessity of giving you this news, thus abruptly, but I must explain why no one can be allowed to leave this room . . ."

It was an hour later when she finally got to the reception room, and the leather case was gone.

Boone had told her the case contained cylinders he had dictated in his Washington office that afternoon, and that was all she knew. It wasn't remarkable that he hadn't told her what the dictation was about, because he seldom did. Since he used other stenographers for all routine stuff, it was understood that any cylinders he turned over to her personally were important and probably confidential. There were twelve such cases in use in Boone's office, each holding ten cylinders, and they were constantly going back and forth among him and her and other stenographers, since Boone had done nearly all of his dictating on the machine. They were numbered, stamped on top, and this one had been number four. The machine that Boone had used was the Stenophone.

Miss Gunther admitted that she had made a mistake. She had not mentioned the missing case to anyone until Wednesday morning, when the police had asked her what had been in the leather case which she had had with her when she came to the reception room for a cocktail. Some NIA louse had of course told the police about it. She had told the police that she had been ashamed to confess her negligence, and anyway her silence had done no harm, since the case could have had no connection with the murder.

"Four people," Wolfe murmured, "say that you took the case with you from the reception room to the ballroom."

Phoebe Gunther nodded, unimpressed. She was drinking Bourbon and water and smoking a cigarette. "You believe them or you believe me. It wouldn't surprise me if four of that kind of people said they looked through the keyhole and saw me kill Mr. Boone. Or even forty."

"You mean NIA people. But Mrs. Boone isn't one."

"No," Phoebe agreed. She lifted her shoulders, kept them up a second, and let them down. "Mr. Kates told me what she said. Mrs. Boone doesn't like me. Yet—I rather doubt if that's true—I think maybe she does like me, but she hated having her husband depend on me. You notice she didn't actually lie about it; she didn't say she saw me have the case when I left the reception room."

"What did Mr. Boone depend on you for?"

"To do what he told me to."

"Of course." Wolfe was merely murmuring. "But what did he get from you? Intelligent obedience? Loyalty? Comfortable companionship? Happiness? Ecstasy?"

"Oh, for the lord's sake." She looked mildly disgusted. "You sound like a congressman's wife. What he got was first-class work. I'm not saying that during the two years I worked for Mr. Boone I was always fresh out of ecstasy, but I never took it to the office with me, and anyway I was saving it up until I met Mr. Goodwin." She gestured. "You've been reading old-fashioned novels too. If you want to know whether I was on terms of sinful intimacy with Mr. Boone, the answer is no. For one thing, he was too busy, and so was I, and anyhow he didn't strike me that way. I merely worshiped him."

"You did?"

"Yes, I did." She gave the impression that she meant it. "He was irritable and he expected too much, he was overweight and he had dandruff, and he nearly drove me crazy trying to keep his schedule under control, but he was honest clear through and the best man in Washington, and he was up against the dirtiest gang of pigs and chiselers on earth. So since I was born weak-minded to begin with, I merely worshiped him, but where he was getting ecstasy I really don't know."

That would seem to cover the ecstasy angle. It was around that point, as I filled page after page in my notebook, that I took a sounding on how much of it I believed, and when I found my credibility gauge mounting up into the nineties and still ascending, I disqualified myself for bias.

She had a definite opinion about the murder. She doubted if any number of NIA members were in cahoots on it, probably not even two of them, because they were too cagey to conspire to commit a murder that would be a nation-wide sensation. Her idea was that some one member had done it himself or hired it done, and it had to be one whose interests had been so damaged or threatened by Boone that he was willing to disregard the black eye the NIA would get. She accepted Wolfe's theory that it was now desirable, from the standpoint of the NIA, that the murderer be caught.

"Then doesn't it follow," Wolfe asked, "that you and the BPR would prefer not to have him caught?"

"It may follow," she admitted. "But I'm afraid that personally I'm not that logical, so I don't feel that way."

"Because you worshiped Mr. Boone? That's understandable. But in that case, why didn't you accept my invitation to come and discuss it last evening?"

She either had it ready or didn't need to get it ready. "Because I didn't feel like it. I was tired and I didn't know who would be here. Between the police and the FBI, I have answered a thousand questions a thousand times each and I needed a rest."

"But you came with Mr. Goodwin."

"Certainly. Any girl who needed a rest would go anywhere with Mr. Goodwin, because she wouldn't have to use her mind." She didn't even toss me a glance, but went on, "However, I didn't intend to stay all night, and it's after two, and what about my turn?"

That was when Wolfe looked at the clock and sighed and told her to go ahead.

She shifted in the chair to change pressure, took a couple of sips from her glass and put it down, leaned her head back against the red leather, getting a very nice effect, and asked as if it didn't matter much one way or the other:

"Who approached you from the NIA, what did they say, what have you agreed to do, and how much are they paying you?"

Wolfe was so startled he almost blinked at her. "Oh, no, Miss Gunther, nothing like that."

"Why not?" she demanded. "Then it wasn't a bargain at all."

He considered, realizing what he had let himself in for. "Very well," he said, "let's see. Mr. Erskine and his son, and Mr. Breslow and Mr. Winterhoff came to see me. Later Mr. O'Neill also came. They said many things, but the upshot was that they hired me to investigate. I have agreed to do so and to attempt to catch the murderer. What—"

"No matter who it is?"

"Yes. Don't interrupt. What they pay will depend on the expenses incurred and what I decide to charge. It will be adequate. I don't like the NIA. I'm an anarchist."

He had decided to make the best of it by being whimsical. She ignored that.

"Did they try to persuade you that the murderer is not an NIA member?"

"No."

"Did you get the impression that they suspect any particular person?"

"No."

"Do you think one of the five who came to see you committed the murder?"

"No."

"Do you mean you are satisfied that none of them did commit it?"

"No."

She made a gesture. "This is silly. You aren't playing fair. You say nothing but no."

"I'm answering your questions. And so far I haven't told you a lie. I doubt if you could say as much."

"Why, what did I tell you that wasn't true?"

"I have no idea. Not yet. I will have. Go ahead."

I broke in, to Wolfe. "Excuse me, but I have no precedent for this, you being grilled by a murder suspect. Am I supposed to take it down?"

He ignored me and repeated to her, "Go ahead. Mr. Goodwin was merely making an opportunity to call you a murder suspect."

She was concentrating and also ignored me. "Do you think," she asked, "that the use of the monkey wrench, which no one could have known would be there, proves that the murder was unpremeditated?"

"No."

"Why not?"

"Because the murderer could have come armed, have seen the wrench, and decided to use it instead."

"But it might have been unpremeditated?"

"Yes."

"Has any NIA man said anything to you that indicated that he or any of them might know who took that leather case or what happened to it?"

"No."

"Or where it is now?"

"No."

"Have you any idea who the murderer is?"

"No."

"Why did you send Mr. Goodwin after me? Why me, instead of—oh, anyone?"

"Because you had stayed away and I wanted to find out why."

She stopped, sat erect, sipped at her glass again, draining it, and brushed her hair back.

"This is a lot of nonsense," she said emphatically. "I could go on asking you questions for hours, and how would I know that a single thing you told me was the truth? For instance, I would give I don't know what for that case. You say that as far as you know no one knows what happened to it or where it is, and it may be in this room right now, there in your desk." She looked at the glass, saw it was empty, and put it down on the check-writing table.

Wolfe nodded. "That is always the difficulty. I was under the same handicap with you."

"But I have nothing to lie about!"

"Pfui. Everybody has something to lie about. Go ahead."

"No." She stood up and saw to her skirt. "It's perfectly useless. I'll go home and go to bed. Look at me. Do I look like a played-out hag?"

That startled him again. His attitude toward women was such that they rarely asked him what they looked like.

He muttered, "No."

"But I am," she declared. "That's the way it always affects me. The tireder I get the less I look it. Tuesday I got the hardest blow I ever got in my life, and since then I haven't had a decent night's sleep, and look at me." She turned to me. "Would you mind showing me which way to go for a taxi?"

"I'll run you up," I told her. "I have to put the car away anyhow."

She told Wolfe good night, and we got our things on and went out and climbed in. She let her head fall back against the cushion and closed her eyes for a second, then opened them, straightened up, and flashed a glance at me.

"So you took Nero Wolfe on," I remarked, as to a comparative stranger.

"Don't be aloof," she said. She reached to put her fingers around my arm, three inches below the shoulder, and press. "Don't pay any attention to that. It doesn't mean anything. Once in a while I like to feel a man's arm, that's all."

"Okay, I'm a man."

"So I suspected."

"When this is all over I'd be glad to teach you how to play pool or look up words in the dictionary."

"Thanks." I thought she shivered. "When this is all over."

When we stopped for a light in the upper Forties she said, "You know, I believe I'm going to be hysterical. But don't pay any attention to that either."

I looked at her, and there certainly wasn't any sign of it

in her voice or her face. I never saw anyone act less hysterical. When I pulled up at the curb at her address, she hopped out before I could move and stuck her hand in.

"Good night. Or what is the protocol? Does a detective shake hands with one of the suspects?"

"Sure." We shook. It fitted nicely ."To get her off her guard."

She disappeared inside, probably to give the doorman a brief glance on her way to the elevator, to strengthen his motive.

When I got back home, after putting the car away, and stopped in the office to make sure the safe was locked, there was a scribbled note lying on my desk:

> Archie: Do not communicate further with Miss Gunther except on my order. A woman who is not a fool is dangerous. I don't like this case and shall decide tomorrow whether to abandon it and refund the retainer. In the morning get Panzer and Gore here. NW

Which gave me a rough idea of the state of confusion he was in, the way the note contradicted itself. Saul Panzer's rate was thirty bucks a day, and Bill Gore's was twenty, not to mention expenses, and his committing himself to such an outlay was absolute proof that there would be no retainer refund. He was merely appealing for my sympathy because he had taken on such a hard job. I went up two flights to my room, glancing at the door of his as I passed it on the first landing, and noting that the little red light was on, showing that he had flipped the switch for the alarm connection.

12.

I REALIZED all the more how hard the job was likely to be when, the next morning after Wolfe came down from the plant rooms at eleven o'clock, I heard him giving Saul Panzer and Bill Gore their instructions.

To anyone seeing him but not knowing him, Saul Panzer was nothing but a little guy with a big nose who never quite caught up with his shaving. To the few who knew him, Wolfe and me for instance, those details meant nothing. He was the one free-lance operative in New York who, year in and year out, always had at least ten times more jobs offered him than he had the time or inclination to take. He never turned Wolfe down if he could possibly help it. That morning he sat with his old brown cap on his knee, taking no notes because he never had to, while Wolfe described the situation and told him to spend as many hours or days at the Waldorf as might be necessary, milking and gathering eggs. He was to cover everything and everybody.

Bill Gore was full size and unpolished, and one glance at the top of his head showed that he was doomed. He would be bald in another five years. His immediate objective was the NIA office, where he was to compile certain lists and records. Erskine had been phoned to and had promised cooperation.

After they had departed I asked Wolfe, "Is it really as bad as that?"

He frowned at me. "As bad as what?"

"You know darned well what. Fifty dollars a day for the dregs. Where is there any genius in that?"

"Genius?" His frown became a scowl. "What can genius do with this confounded free-for-all? A thousand people, all with motive and opportunity, and the means at hand! Why the devil I ever let you persuade me—"

"No, sir," I said loudly and firmly. "Don't try it! When I saw how tough this was going to be, and then when I read that note you left for me last night, it was obvious you would try to blame it on me. Nothing doing. I admit I didn't know how desperate it was until I heard you telling Saul and Bill to dive into the holes the cops have already cleaned out. You don't have to admit you're licked. You can wriggle out. I'll draw a check to the NIA for their ten thousand, and you can dictate a letter to them saying that on account of having caught the mumps, or perhaps it would be better—"

"Shut up," he growled. "How can I return money I haven't received?"

"But you have. The check was in the morning mail and I've deposited it."

"Good God. It's in the bank?"

"Yes, sir."

He pushed the button, savagely, for beer. He was as close to being in a panic as I remembered seeing him.

"So you have nothing," I said without mercy. "Nothing whatever?"

"Certainly I have something."

"Yeah? What?"

"Something Mr. O'Neill said yesterday afternoon. Something very peculiar."

"What?"

He shook his head. "Not for you. I'll put Saul or Bill on it tomorrow."

I didn't believe a word of it. For ten minutes I went over in my mind everything I remembered Don O'Neill saying, and then believed it less than ever.

All day Saturday he had no jobs for me connected with the Boone case, not even a phone call to make. The calls all came the other way, and there were plenty of those. Most of them, from newspapers and Cramer's office and so on, were nothing but blah. Two of them were merely comic relief:

Winterhoff, the Man of Distinction, phoned around noon. He wanted something for his money right away. The cops were after him. Many hours of questioning about fourteen people had got it settled that it was he who had suggested the little room near the stage for Boone's privacy and had escorted him there, and he was being harassed. He had explained that his knowledge of the room had come from his participation in previous affairs on those premises, but they weren't satisfied. He wanted Wolfe to certify to his innocence and instruct the police to let him alone. His order wasn't filled.

Just before lunch there was a call from a man with an educated voice who said his name was Adamson, of counsel for the NIA. His tone implied that he wasn't very crazy about Wolfe's being hired anyway, and he wanted practically everything, including a daily report of all activities, operations, conversations, contacts, and intentions. He insisted on speaking to Wolfe, which was a mistake on his part, because if he had been willing to talk with me I might at least have treated him with common courtesy.

Another thing the NIA wanted the very day we got their retainer check was something we couldn't have furnished even if we had felt like it. This request was brought by their Hattie Harding in person, in the middle of the afternoon, just after Wolfe went up to the orchids. I took her to the office and we sat on the couch. She was still well put together and well dressed, and her eyes were still competent, but the strain was telling on her. She looked much nearer forty-eight than twenty-six.

She had come to yell for help, though she didn't put it that way. To hear her tell it, there was hell to pay from coast to coast and the end of the world was expected any minute. Public Relations was on its last legs. Hundreds of telegrams were pouring into the NIA office, from members and friends all over the country, telling of newspaper editorials, of resolutions passed by Chambers of Commerce and all sorts of clubs and groups, and of talk in the street. Even—this was strictly off the record—eleven resignations had been received from members, one a member of the Board of Directors. Something had to be done.

I asked what.

Something, she said.

"Like catching the murderer?"

"That, of course." She seemed to regard that as a mere detail. "But something to stop this insane hullabaloo. Perhaps a statement signed by a hundred prominent citizens. Or telegrams urging sermons tomorrow—tomorrow is Sunday—"

"Are you suggesting that Mr. Wolfe should send telegrams to fifty thousand preachers and priests and rabbis?"

"No, of course not." Her hands fluttered. "But something—something—"

"Listen, P.R." I patted her on the knee to quiet her. "You are stricken, I appreciate that. But the NIA seems to think this is a department store. Who you want is not Nero Wolfe but Russell Birdwell or Eddie Bernays. This is a specialty shop. All we're going to do is catch the murderer."

"Oh, my God," she said. Then she added, "I doubt it."

"Doubt what?" I stared at her. "That we're going to catch him?"

"Yes. That anyone is."

"Why?"

"I just doubt it." She met my gaze, competently. Then her eyes changed. "Look, this is off the record?"

"Sure, you and me. And my boss, but he never tells anybody anything."

"I'm fed up." She worked her jaw like a man, no lip trembling. "I'm going to quit and get a job sewing on buttons. The day anyone catches the murderer of Cheney Boone, finds him and proves it on him, it will rain up instead of down. In fact it will—"

I nodded encouragingly. "What else will it do?"

She abruptly got to her feet. "I'm talking too much."

"Oh, no, not enough. You've just started. Sit down."

"No, thank you." Her eyes were competent again. "You're the first man I've collapsed in front of for a long, long time. For heaven's sake, don't get the idea that I know secrets and try to dig them out of me. It's just that this thing is more than I can handle and I've lost my head. Don't bother to let me out."

She went.

When Wolfe came down to the office at six o'clock I reported the conversation in full. At first he decided not to be interested, then changed his mind. He wanted my opinion and

I gave it to him, that I doubted if she knew anything that would help much, and even if she did she was through collapsing in front of me, but he might have a go at her.

He grunted. "Archie. You are transparent. What you mean is that you don't want to bother with her, and you don't want to bother with her because Miss Gunther has got you fidgeting."

I said coldly, " I don't fidget."

"Miss Gunther has got you on a string."

Usually I stay right with him when he takes that line, but there was no telling how far he might go in the case of Phoebe Gunther and I didn't want to resign in the middle of a murder job, so I cut it off by going to the front door for the evening papers.

We get two of each, to avoid friction, and I handed him his share and sat at my desk with mine. I looked at the *Gazette* first, and on the front page saw headlines that looked like news. It was. Mrs. Boone had got something in the mail.

One detail that I believe I haven't mentioned before was Boone's wallet. I haven't mentioned it because its being taken by the murderer provided no new angle on the crime or the motive, since he hadn't carried money in it. His money had been in a billfold in his hip pocket and hadn't been touched. He had carried the wallet in the breast pocket of his coat and used it for miscellaneous papers and cards, and it had not been found on the body, and therefore it was presumed that the murderer had taken it. The news in the *Gazette* was that Mrs. Boone had received an envelope in the mail that morning, with her name and address printed on it with a lead pencil, and in it had been two objects that Boone had always carried in the wallet: his automobile license and a photograph of Mrs. Boone in her wedding dress. The *Gazette* article remarked that the sender must be both a sentimentalist and a realist; sentimental, because the photo was returned; realist, because the auto license, which was still of use, had been returned, while Boone's operator's license, which he had also kept in the wallet, had not been. The *Gazette* writer was picturesque about it, saying that the operator's license had been canceled with a monkey wrench.

"Indeed," Wolfe said loud enough for me to hear. I saw that he was reading it too, and spoke:

"If the cops hadn't already been there and got it, and if Miss Gunther didn't have me on a string, I'd run up to see Mrs. Boone and get that envelope."

"Three or four men in a laboratory," Wolfe said, "will do everything to that envelope but split its atoms. Before long they'll be doing that too. But this is the first finger that has pointed in any direction at all."

"Sure," I agreed, "now it's a cinch. All we have to do is find out which of those one thousand four hundred and ninety-two people is both a sentimentalist and a realist, and we've got him."

We went back to our papers.

Nothing more before dinner. After the meal, which for me consisted chiefly of thin toast and liver paté on account of the way Fritz makes the pâté, we had just got back to the office again, a little before nine, when a telegram came. I took it from the envelope and handed it to Wolfe, and after he had read it he passed it over to me. It ran:

NERO WOLFE 922 WEST 35 NYC
CIRCUMSTANCES MAKE IT IMPOSSIBLE TO CONTINUE SURVEILLANCE OF ONEILL BUT BELIEVE IT ESSENTIAL THIS BE DONE ALTHOUGH CAN GUARANTEE NOTHING
BRESLOW

I put my brows up at Wolfe. He was looking at me with his eyes half open, which meant he was really looking.

"Perhaps," he said witheringly, "you will be good enough to tell me what other arrangements you have made for handling this case without my knowledge?"

I grinned at him. "No, sir. Not me. I was about to ask if you have put Breslow on the payroll and if so at how much, so I can enter it."

"You know nothing of this?"

"No. Don't you?"

"Get Mr. Breslow on the phone."

That wasn't so simple. We knew only that Breslow was a manufacturer of paper products from Denver, and that, having come to New York for the NIA meeting, he was staying on, as a member of the Executive Committee, to help hold the fort in the crisis. I knew Frank Thomas Erskine was at the Churchill and tried that, but he was out. Hattie Harding's number, which was in the phone book, gave me a don't answer signal. So I tried Lon Cohen again at the *Gazette*, which I should have done in the first place, and learned that Breslow was at the Strider-Weir. In another three minutes I had him and switched him to Wolfe, but kept myself connected.

He sounded on the phone just the way he looked, red-faced with anger.

"Yes, Wolfe? Have you got something? Well? Well?"

"I have a question to ask—"

"Yes? What is it?"

"I am about to ask it. That was why I had Mr. Goodwin

learn your number, and call it and ask for you, so you could be on one end of the telephone and me on the other end, and then I could ask you this question. Tell me when you are ready, sir."

"I'm ready! Damn it, what is it?"

"Good. Here it is. About that telegram you sent me—"

"Telegram? What telegram? I haven't sent you any telegram!"

"You know nothing about a telegram to me?"

"No! Nothing whatever! What—"

"Then it's a mistake. They must have got the name wrong. I suspected as much. I was expecting one from a man named Bristow. I apologize, sir, for disturbing you. Good-by."

Breslow tried to prolong the agony, but between us we got him off.

"So," I remarked, "he didn't send it. If he did, and didn't want us to know it, why would he sign his name? Do we have it traced? Or do we save energy by assuming that whoever sent it knows about phone booths?"

"Confound it," Wolfe said bitterly. "Probably someone peddling herrings. But we can't afford to ignore it." He glanced at the wall clock, which said three minutes past nine. "Find out if Mr. O'Neill is at home. Just ask him—no. Let me have him."

The number of O'Neill's residence, an apartment on Park Avenue, was listed, and I got both it and him. Wolfe took it, and told him about the request from Adamson, the NIA lawyer, and fed him a long rigmarole about the inadvisability of written reports. O'Neill said he didn't care a hang about reports, written or otherwise, and they parted friends.

Wolfe considered a moment. "No. We'll let him go for tonight. You had better get him in the morning as he leaves. If we decide to keep it up we can get Orrie Cather."

13.

TAILING as a solo job in New York can be almost anything, depending on the circumstances. You can wear out your brain and muscles in a strenuous ten-hour stretch, keeping contact only by using all the dodges on the list and inventing some more as you go along, and then lose him by some lousy little break that nothing and no one could have prevented. Or you can lose him the first five minutes, especially if he knows you're there. Or, also in the first five minutes, he can take to a chair somewhere, an office or a hotel room, and stay there all day, not giving a damn how bored you get.

So you never know, but what I fully expected was a long day of nothing, since it was Sunday. A little after eight in the morning I sat in a taxi which, headed downtown, was parked on Park Avenue in the Seventies, fifty paces north of the entrance to the apartment house where O'Neill lived. I would have given even money that I would still be there six hours later, or even twelve, though I admitted there was a fair chance of our going to church at eleven, or to a restaurant for two o'clock dinner. I couldn't even read the Sunday paper with any satisfaction because I had to keep my eye on the entrance. The taxi driver was my old stand-by Herb Aronson, but he had never seen O'Neill. As the time went by we discussed various kinds of matters, and he read aloud to me from the *Times*.

At ten o'clock we decided to get a bet down. Each of us would write on a slip of paper the time that we thought my man would stick his nose out, and the one that was furthest off would pay the other one a cent a minute for the time he missed it by. Herb was just handing me a scrap he tore from the *Times* for me to write my guess on when I saw Don O'Neill emerging to the sidewalk.

I told Herb, "Save it for next time. That's him."

Whatever O'Neill did, it would be awkward, because his doorman knew us by heart by that time. He had previously signaled to Herb for a customer, and Herb had turned him down. What O'Neill did was look toward us, with me keeping my face in a corner so he couldn't see it if his vision was good for that distance, and speak to the doorman, who shook his head. That was about as awkward as it could get, unless O'Neill had walked to us for a conference.

Herb told me out of the corner of his mouth, "Our strategy stinks. He takes a taxi and we ride his tail, and when he comes home the doorman tells him he's being followed."

"So what was I to do?" I demanded. "Disguise myself as a flower girl and stand at the corner selling daffodils? Next time you plan it. This whole tailing idea has got to be a joke. Start your engine. Anyhow, he'll never get home. We'll pinch him for murder before the day's out. Start your engine! He's getting transportation."

The doorman had been blowing his whistle, and a taxi on its way south had swerved and was stopping at the curb. The doorman opened the door and O'Neill got in, and the taxi slid away. Herb got into gear and we moved.

"This," Herb said, "is the acme. The absolute acme. Why don't we just pull up to him and ask where he's going?"

"Because," I said, "you don't know an acme when you see one. He has no reason at all to think we're following him unless he has been alerted, and in that case nothing would unalert him and we are lost. Keep back a little more—just enough not to let a light part us."

Herb did so, and managed the light stops as if his heart was in it. With the thin traffic of Sunday morning, there were only two of them before we got to Forty-sixth Street, where O'Neill's cab turned left. One block over, at Lexington Avenue, it turned right, and in another minute it had stopped at the entrance to Grand Central Station.

We were two cars behind. Herb swung to the right and braked, and I stepped out behind a parked car and grinned at him. "Didn't I tell you? He's hopping it. See you in court." As soon as O'Neill had paid his driver and started across the sidewalk I left cover.

I was still selling it short. What I would have settled for at that stage was a ride out to Greenwich to join a week-end party for some drinks and maybe poker. At any rate, O'Neill didn't seem to be in any doubt as to what he would settle for, for he marched down the long corridor and across the concourse of the station like a man with a destination. He gave no sign of suspecting that anyone had an eye on him. Where he finally wound up was not one of the train entrances, but the main parcel room on the upper level. I lingered at a distance, with a corner handy. There were several ahead of him and he waited his turn, then handed in a ticket, and in a minute or so was given an object.

Even from where I stood, about thirty feet off, the object looked as if it might be of interest. It was a little rectangular leather case. He grabbed it up and went. I was now somewhat less interested in keeping my presence undetected, but a lot more interested in not losing him, so I closed up some, and nearly stepped on his heels when he suddenly slowed up, almost to a stop, put the case inside his topcoat, got his arm snugly around it, and buttoned the coat. Then he went on. Instead of returning to the Lexington Avenue entrance he went up the ramp toward Forty-second Street, and when he got to the sidewalk turned left, to where the taxis stop in front of the Commodore Hotel. He still hadn't spotted me. After a short wait he snared a cab, opened the door and got in, and reached to pull the door shut.

I decided that would not do. It would have been nice to know what address he would give the driver if there were no interruptions, but that wasn't vital, whereas if I lost contact with that leather case through the hazards of solo tailing I would have to get a job helping Hattie Harding sew on buttons. So I moved fast enough to use a hand to keep the door from closing and spoke:

"Hello there, Mr. O'Neill! Going uptown? Mind giving me a lift?"

I was on the seat beside him, and now, willing to do my share, pulled the door shut.

I am not belittling him when I say he was flustered. It would have flustered most men. And he did pretty well.

"Why, hello, Goodwin! Where did you come from? I'm—well, no, the fact is I'm not going uptown. I'm going downtown."

"Make up your mind," the driver growled through at us.

"It doesn't matter," I told O'Neill cheerfully. "I just want to ask you a couple of questions about that leather case that's under your coat." I said to the driver, "Go ahead. Turn south on Eighth."

The driver was glaring at me. "It's not your cab. What is this, a hard touch?"

"No," O'Neill told him. "It's all right. We're friends. Go ahead."

The cab moved. There was no conversation. We passed Vanderbilt and, after waiting for a light, were crossing Madison when O'Neill leaned forward to tell the driver:

"Turn north on Fifth Avenue."

The driver was too hurt to reply, but when we got to Fifth and had a green light he turned right. I said:

"All right if you want to, but I thought we would save time by going straight to Nero Wolfe's place. He will be even curiouser than I am about what's in that thing. Of course we shouldn't discuss it in this taxi, since the driver doesn't like us."

He leaned forward again and gave the driver his home address on Park Avenue. I thought that over for three blocks and voted against it. The only weapon I had on me was a penknife. Since I had been watching that entrance since eight o'clock it was unlikely that the NIA Executive Committee was assembled in O'Neill's apartment, but if they were, and especially if General Erskine was with them, it would require too much exertion on my part to walk out of there with that case. So I spoke to O'Neill in an undertone:

"Lookit. If he's a public-spirited citizen, and if he hears anything that gives him the idea this is connected with murder, he'll probably stop at the first cop he sees. Maybe that's what you want too, a cop. If so you will be glad to know that I don't like the idea of your apartment and if we go there I'll display a license to that doorman, put my arms around you, and make him call the Nineteenth Precinct, which is at 153 East Sixty-seventh Street, Rhinelander four, one-four-four-five. That would create a hubbub. Why not get rid of this eavesdropper and talk it over on a bench in the sunshine? Also I saw the look in your eye and don't try it. I'm more than twenty years younger than you and I do exercises every morning."

He relinquished the expression of a tiger about to leap and leaned forward to tell the driver:

"Stop here."

Although I doubted if he carried shooters, I didn't want him fooling around his pockets, so I settled with the meter myself. We were at Sixty-ninth Street. After the cab had rolled off we crossed the avenue, walked to one of the benches against the wall enclosing Central Park, and sat down. He was keeping his left arm hooked tight around the object under his coat.

I said, "One easy way would be for me to take a look at it, inside and out. If it contains only black market butter, God bless you."

He turned sideways to regard me as man to man. "I'll tell you, Goodwin." He was choosing his words. "I'm not going to try a lot of stuff like indignation about your following me and that kind of stuff." I thought he wasn't choosing very well, repeating himself, but I was too polite to interrupt. "But I can explain how I happen to have this case, absolutely innocently—absolutely! And I don't know any more than you do about what's in it—I have no idea!"

"Let's look and see."

"No." He was firm. "As far as you know, it's my property—"

"But is it?"

"As far as you know it is, and I have a right to examine it privately. I mean a moral right, I admit I can't put it on the ground of legal right because you have offered to refer it to the police and that is of course legally correct. But I do have the moral right. You first suggested that we should go with it to Nero Wolfe. Do you think the police would approve of that?"

"No, but he would."

"I don't doubt it." O'Neill was in his stride now, earnest and persuasive. "But you see, neither of us actually wants to go to the police. Actually our interests coincide. It's merely a question of procedure. Look at it from your personal angle: what you want is to be able to go to your employer and say to him, 'You sent me to do a job, and I have done it, and here are the results,' and then deliver this leather case to him, and me right there with you if you want it that way. Isn't that what you want?"

"Sure. Let's go."

"We will go. I assure you, Goodwin, we will go." He was so sincere it was almost painful. "But does it matter exactly *when* we go? Now or four hours from now? Of course it doesn't! I have never broken a promise in my life. I'm a businessman, and the whole basis of American business is integrity—absolute integrity. That brings us back to my moral rights in this matter. What I propose is this: I will go to my office, at 1270 Sixth Avenue. You will come there for me at three o'clock, or I will meet you anywhere you say, and I will have this leather case with me, and we will take it to Nero Wolfe."

"I don't—"

"Wait. Whatever my moral rights may be, if you extend me this courtesy you deserve to have it acknowledged and appreciated. When I meet you at three o'clock I will hand you one thousand dollars in currency as evidence of appreciation. A point I didn't mention: I will guarantee that Wolfe will know nothing about this four-hour delay. That will be easy to arrange. If I had the thousand dollars with me I would give it to you now. I have never broken a promise in my life."

I looked at my wrist and appealed to him, "Make it ten thousand."

He wasn't staggered, but only grieved, and he wasn't even grieved beyond endurance. "That's out of the question," he declared, but not in a tone to give offense. "Absolutely out of the question. One thousand is the limit."

I grinned at him. "It would be fun to see how far up I could get you, but it's ten minutes to eleven, so in ten minutes Mr. Wolfe will come down to his office and I don't like to keep him waiting. The trouble is it's Sunday and I never take bribes on Sunday. Forget it. Here are the alternatives: You and I and the object under your coat go now to Mr. Wolfe. Or give me the object and I take it to him, and you go for a walk or take a nap. Or I yell at that cop across the street and tell him to call the precinct, which I admit I like least, but you've got your moral rights. Heretofore I've been in no hurry, but now Mr. Wolfe will be downstairs, so I give you two minutes."

He wanted to try. "Four hours! That's all! I'll make it five thousand, and you come with me and I'll give it to you—"

"No. Forget it. Didn't I say it's Sunday? Come on, hand it over."

"I am not going to let this case out my sight."

"Okay." I got up and crossed to the curb and stood so as to keep one eye out for a taxi and one on him. Before long I flagged an empty and it turned in to me and stopped. It had probably been years since Don O'Neill had done anything he disapproved of as strongly as he did of arising and walking to the cab and getting in, but he made it. I dropped beside him and gave the driver the address.

14.

TEN hollow black cylinders, about three inches in diameter and six inches long, stood on end in two neat rows on Wolfe's desk. Beside them, with the lid open, was the case, of good heavy leather, somewhat battered and scuffed. On the outside of the lid a big figure four was stamped. On its inside a label was pasted:

BUREAU OF PRICE REGULATION
POTOMAC BUILDING
WASHINGTON D.C.

Before pasting in the label someone had typed on it in caps: OFFICE OF CHENEY BOONE, DIRECTOR.

I was at my desk and Wolfe was at his. Don O'Neill was walking up and down with his hands in his pants pockets. The atmosphere was not hail fellow well met. I had given Wolfe a full report, including O'Neill's last-minute offer to me of five grand, and Wolfe's self-esteem was such that he always regarded any attempt to buy me off as a personal affront, not to me but to him. I have often wondered who he would blame if I sold out once, himself or me.

He had repudiated without discussion O'Neill's claim to a moral right to hear what was on the cylinders before anyone else, and when O'Neill had seen it was hopeless the look on his face was such that I had decided to make sure and had given him a good frisking. He was not packing any tools, but that had not improved the atmosphere. The question then arose, how were we to make the cylinders perform? The next day, a business day, it would have been easy, but this was Sunday. It was O'Neill who solved the problem. The President of the Stenophone Company was a member of the NIA and O'Neill knew him. He lived in Jersey. O'Neill phoned him and, without disclosing any incriminating details, got him to phone the manager of his New York office and showroom, who lived in Brooklyn, and instruct him to go to the showroom, get a

Stenophone and bring it to Wolfe's office. That was what we were sitting there waiting for—that is, Wolfe and I were sitting and O'Neill was walking.

"Mr. O'Neill." Wolfe opened his eyes enough to see. "That tramping back and forth is extremely irritating."

"I'm not going to leave this room," O'Neill declared without halting.

"Shall I tie him up?" I offered.

Wolfe, ignoring me, told O'Neill, "It will probably be another hour or more. What about your statement that you got possession of this thing innocently? Your word. Do you want to explain that now? How you got it innocently?"

"I'll explain it when I feel like it."

"Nonsense. I didn't take you for a nincompoop."

"Go to hell."

That always annoyed Wolfe. He said sharply, "Then you are a nincompoop. You have only two means of restraining Mr. Goodwin and me: your own physical prowess or an appeal to the police. The former is hopeless; Mr. Goodwin could fold you up and put you on a shelf. You obviously don't like the idea of the police, I can't imagine why, since you're innocent. So how do you like this: when that machine has arrived and we have learned how to run it and the manager has departed, Mr. Goodwin will carry you out and set you on the stoop, and come back in and shut the door. Then he and I will listen to the cylinders."

O'Neill stopped walking, took his hands from his pockets and put them flat on the desk to lean on them, and glowered at Wolfe.

"You won't do that!"

"I won't. Mr. Goodwin will."

"Damn you!" He held the pose long enough for five takes, then slowly straightened up. "What do you want?"

"I want to know where you got this thing."

"All right, I'll tell you. Last evening—"

"Excuse me. Archie. Your notebook. Go ahead, sir."

"Last evening around eight-thirty I got a phone call at home. It was a woman. She said her name was Dorothy Unger and she was a stenographer at the New York office of the Bureau of Price Regulation. She said she had made a bad mistake. She said that in an envelope addressed to me she had enclosed something that was supposed to be enclosed in a letter to someone else. She said that she had remembered about it after she got home, and that she might even lose her job if her boss found out about it. She asked me when I received the envelope to mail the enclosure to her at her home, and she gave me her address. I asked her what the enclosure was and she said it was a ticket for a parcel that had been checked at Grand Central Station. I asked her some more questions and told her I would do what she asked me to."

Wolfe put in, "Of course you phoned her back."

"I couldn't. She said she had no phone and was calling from a booth. This morning I received the envelope and the enclosure was—"

"This is Sunday," Wolfe snapped.

"Damn it, I know it's Sunday! It came special delivery. It contained a circular about price ceilings, and the enclosure. If it had been a weekday I would have communicated with the BPR office, but of course the office wasn't open." O'Neill gestured impatiently. "What does it matter what I would have done or what I thought? You know what I did do. Naturally, you know more about it than me, since you arranged the whole thing!"

"I see." Wolfe put up a brow. "You think I arranged it?"

"No." O'Neill leaned on the desk again. "I *know* you arranged it! What happened? Wasn't Goodwin right there? I admit I was dumb when I came here Friday. I was afraid you had agreed to frame Boone's murder on someone in the BPR, or at least someone outside the NIA. And already, you must have been, you were preparing to frame someone *in* the NIA! Me! No wonder you think I'm a nincompoop!"

He jerked erect, glared at Wolfe, turned to glare at me, went to the red leather chair and sat down, and said in a completely different voice, calm and controlled:

"But you'll find that I'm not a nincompoop."

"That point," Wolfe said, frowning at him, "is relatively unimportant. The envelope you received this morning special delivery—have you got it with you?"

"No."

"Where is it, at your home?"

"Yes."

"Telephone and tell someone to bring it here."

"No. I'm going to have some detective work done on that envelope and not by you."

"Then you won't hear what those cylinders have to say," Wolfe explained patiently. "Must I keep repeating that?"

This time O'Neill didn't try to argue. He used the phone on my desk, dialed, got his party, and told someone whom he called Honey to get the envelope as described from the top of his chiffonier and send it by messenger to Nero Wolfe's office. I was surprised. I would have made it five to one that there was no such envelope, and it was still even money with me that it would be gone from the chiffonier because it must have dropped to the floor and the maid thought it was trash.

When O'Neill was back in the red leather chair Wolfe said, "You're going to find it a little difficult to get anyone to believe that you suspect Mr. Goodwin and me of arranging this. For if that's true, why didn't you insist on going to the police? He wanted to."

"He did not want to." O'Neill was keeping calm. "He merely threatened to."

"But the threat worked. Why did it work?"

"You know damn well why it worked. Because I wanted to hear what's on those cylinders."

"You did indeed. Up to five thousand dollars. Why?"

"Do I have to tell you why?"

"No. You don't have to. You know how it stands."

O'Neill gulped. He had probably swallowed "Go to hell" thirty times in thirty minutes. "Because I have reason to suppose, and so have you, that they are confidential dictation by Cheney Boone, and they may have something to do with what happened to him, and if so I want to know it."

Wolfe shook his head reproachfully. "You're inconsistent. Day before yesterday, sitting in that same chair, your attitude was that you of the NIA had nothing to do with it and it was none of your business. Another thing: you didn't try to bribe Mr. Goodwin to let you hear the cylinders. You tried to bribe him to give you four hours alone with them. Were you trying to scoop all of us—the police, the FBI, and me?"

"Yes, I was, if you want to call it scoop. I didn't trust you before, and now . . ."

Now, from his tone, we were something scraped off the under side of a bridge.

I could report it all, since it's still in the notebook, but it isn't worth it. Wolfe decided, apparently more to kill time than anything else, to put the microscope on the episode of the phone call from Dorothy Unger and the receipt of the envelope. He took O'Neill over it, back and forth and up and down, and O'Neill stayed with him, against his strongest instincts and inclinations, because he knew he had to if he wanted to hear those cylinders. I got so fed up with the repetitions that when the doorbell rang the interruption was welcome in more ways than one.

O'Neill sprang from his chair and came along to the front door. On the stoop was a middle-aged square-faced woman in a purple coat. He greeted her as Gretty, took the envelope she handed him, and thanked her.

Back in the office he let Wolfe and me handle it to look it over, but stayed close. It was a regulation BPR envelope, New York office, with his name and home address typed. Right in the corner, over the penalty clause, was a three-cent stamp, and a couple of inches to the left were five more three-cent stamps. Beneath them was printed by hand with a blue pencil: SPECIAL DELIVERY. Inside was a mimeographed BPR circular, dated March 27th, regarding price ceilings on a long list of copper and brass items.

When Wolfe handed it back to O'Neill and he stuck it in his pocket I remarked, "The post-office employees get more careless all the time. With that stamp in the corner canceled and the others not."

"What?" O'Neill got it from his pocket and glared at it. "What of it?"

"Nothing," Wolfe said shortly. "Mr. Goodwin likes to brag. It proves nothing."

I saw no reason why I shouldn't help to kill time, and I resent Wolfe's habit of making personal remarks in front of strangers, especially when he's an enemy, so I was opening my mouth to go on with it when the bell rang again. When I went to answer it O'Neill came along. You might have thought he was training for the job.

It was the Stenophone man. O'Neill did the honors, mentioning the president and apologizing for ruining his Sunday and so on, and I helped with the machine. It didn't amount to much, for O'Neill had explained on the phone that we didn't need a recorder. The chassis of the player had casters, and didn't weigh over sixty pounds anyhow. The Stenophone man wheeled it into the office, and was introduced to Wolfe, and in less than five minutes had us all instructed. Then, since he didn't seem disposed to linger, we let him go.

When I returned to the office after showing the visitor out, Wolfe sent me a certain type of glance to alert me and said:

"Now, Archie, if you'll get Mr. O'Neill's hat and coat, please. He is leaving."

O'Neill stared at him a second and then laughed, or at least made a noise. It was the first downright ugly noise he had made.

Just to try him for size I took two quick steps toward him. He took three quick steps back. I stopped and grinned at him. He tried to look at both Wolfe and me at once.

"So that's how it is," he said, extremely ugly. "You think you can double-cross Don O'Neill. You'd better not."

"Pfui." Wolfe wiggled a finger at him. "I have given you no assurance that you would be permitted to hear these things. It would be manifestly improper to permit an official of the NIA to listen to confidential dictation of the Director of the BPR, even after the Director has been murdered. Besides, you're inconsistent again. A while ago you said you didn't trust me. That could only have been because you considered me untrustworthy. Now you profess to be shocked to find that I am untrustworthy. Utterly inconsistent." The finger wiggled again. "Well, sir? Do you prefer to be self-propelled?"

"I'm not leaving this room."

"Archie?"

I moved to him. This time he didn't budge. From the look on his face, if he had had anything at all useful on him he would have used it. I took him by the arm and said, "Come on, come with Archie. You must weigh a hundred and eighty. I don't want to carry you."

He started a right for my jaw, or at least it seemed that that was what he thought he was doing, but it was too slow to hit anything that wasn't nailed down. Ignoring it, I started to spin him to attach from the rear, and the son of a gun hauled off and kicked me. He tried to kick high and got my knee. I am not claiming that it hurt much, but I do not like kickers. So I plugged him, with my left because it was handiest, on his soft neck just below the ear, and he teetered over against the bookshelves. I supposed that would explain things to him, but he teetered right back and tried another kick, so I used the right with more in it, also to the neck for the sake of knuckles, and he teetered again and tumbled.

I told Wolfe to buzz Fritz to open the door, saw that Fritz was already there, took my fallen foe by the ankles, and dragged him across to the hall, down the hall to the door, and on out to the stoop. Fritz handed me his coat and hat and I dropped them on him, re-entered the hall, and shut the door.

In the office I asked Wolfe, "Is he on the Executive Committee too, or was he just Chairman of the Dinner Committee? I was trying to remember while I was dragging him."

"I dislike commotion," Wolfe said peevishly. "I didn't tell you to hit him."

"He tried to kick me. He did kick me. Next time you do it."

Wolfe shuddered. "Start that machine going."

15.

It took more than an hour altogether to run off the ten cylinders, not counting time out for lunch.

I started the first one at the speed recommended by our instructor, but it had been going only a few seconds when

Wolfe told me to slow it down. Having heard Cheney Boone on the radio I had expected this to sound about the same, but although there was enough similarity to recognize his voice, this seemed to be pitched higher and the words were more distinct. The first one began:

"Six-seventy-nine. Personal. Dear Mr. Pritchard. Thank you very much for your letter but I have decided not to get a Chesapeake retriever but to try an Irish setter. I have nothing against Chesapeakes and there is no good reason for my decision except the unpredictable vagary of the human mind. Sincerely. Six-eighty. Dear Mrs. Ambruster. I do indeed remember that pleasant day and evening in St. Louis last fall and I deeply regret my inability to be present at the spring meeting of your fine organization. The next time I get to St. Louis I shall certainly get in touch with you. The material you request will be sent you without delay, and if it fails to arrive promptly be sure to let me know. With best regards and best wishes for the success of your meeting. Sincerely. Six-eighty-one. Memo—no, make it a letter to all regional directors. By name to each. Please return to this office immediately the advance copies of the press release for March 25th regarding household appliances. That release has been canceled and will not be sent out. Paragraph. The premature disclosure of some of the contents of that release by a press association has again raised the question whether advance copies of releases should be sent to regional offices. You are requested to investigate without delay, in your office, the handling of the advance copies of the release in question, and make a full report of the results directly to me. I shall expect this report to reach me not later than March 28th. Sincerely. Six-eighty-two. Dear Mr. Maspero. Thank you very much for your letter of the 16th, and I assure you that its contents will be regarded as confidential. That of course would be impossible if your information were susceptible of use in a legal action that could be undertaken by me in the performance of my duty, but I am fully aware of the difficulties involved in any attempt . . ."

That one went on long enough to fill at least two full pages single-spaced, leaving room on that cylinder only for two more letters and an interoffice memo. When it reached the end I removed it and returned it to its place in the row, and picked up number two, remarking meanwhile:

"I suppose you noticed that Boone apparently sent his letters by rocket and the regional directors were expected to be streaks of lightning."

Wolfe nodded gloomily. "We've been sniggled." He leaned forward to look at his desk calendar. "He couldn't possibly have dictated that the afternoon of the day he was killed, March 26th. He told the regional directors to investigate and get a report to him by March 28th. Since it was to go to all regional directors, the West Coast was included. Even granting the speed of air mail, and allowing only one day for their investigations, which seems meager, that must have been dictated not later than March 23rd, and probably several days earlier."

He sighed deep. "Confound it. I was hoping—" He compressed his lips and frowned at the leather case. "That woman said four, didn't she?"

"Do you mean Miss Gunther?"

"Who the devil do you think I mean?"

"I think you mean Miss Phoebe Gunther. If so, yes. She said there were twelve of those cases, and the one Boone gave her in the murder room had the number four stamped on top, and he told her it contained cylinders he had dictated in his Washington office that afternoon. So it looks as if someone has been playing button button. Are we too discouraged to go on or would we care to hear number two?"

"Go ahead."

I proceeded with the concert. Lunch intervened at the end of the sixth movement, and after a leisurely but not especially gay meal we returned to the office and finished them up. There was nothing spectacular anywhere in the lot, though some of them contained matter that was certainly confidential; and considered as clues that might help solve a murder. I wouldn't have paid a dime for them. In four others besides number one there was evidence, some of it conclusive, that they had been dictated earlier than March 26th.

I couldn't blame Wolfe for being depressed. In addition to all the other complications, there were at least eight possible explanations of how leather case number four happened, when found, to contain cylinders dictated prior to the day of the murder, the simplest of all being that Boone himself had picked up the wrong case when he left his Washington office that afternoon. Not to mention the basic question, for which I didn't have even a guess, let alone an answer: were the cylinders only a side show or were they part of the main performance?

Leaning back in his chair digesting, Wolfe was, to an unaccustomed eye though not to mine, sound asleep. He didn't stir as I wheeled the machine out of the way, over to a corner. Then, as I went to his desk and started to return the cylinders to their nests in the case, his lids opened to make a slit.

He shook his head. "You'd better run them off again and make a transcription of them. Three carbons." He glanced at the wall clock. "I'll be going upstairs in thirty-five minutes. Do it then."

"Yes, sir." I was grim. "I expected this."

"You did? I didn't."

"I don't mean I expected the cylinders to be antiques. I expected this typewriting job. That's the level this case seems to have descended to."

"Don't badger me. I was an ass to undertake it. I have more Cattleyas than I have room for, and I could have sold five hundred of them for twelve thousand dollars." He let his eyes come half open. "When you have finished transcribing these things, take them down to Mr. Cramer and tell him how we got them."

"Tell him everything?"

"Yes. But before you go to him do another typing job. Your notebook. Send this letter to everyone who was here Friday evening." He frowned for words, and in a moment dictated, " 'Since you were good enough to come to my office at my invitation Friday evening, and since you were present when it was intimated that Miss Gunther's statement that she had left the leather case on the window sill of the reception room might not deserve credence, I am writing to inform you of a development that occurred today. Paragraph. Mr. Don O'Neill received in the mail a ticket for a parcel that had been checked at Grand Central Station. The parcel proved to be the leather case in question, with the figure four stamped on the lid as described by Miss Gunther. However, most of the cylinders it contained were obviously dictated by Mr. Boone prior to March 26th. I send you this information in justice to Miss Gunther.' "

"That's all?" I inquired.

"Yes."

"Cramer will throw a fit."

"No doubt. Mail them before you go to him, and take him a carbon. Then bring Miss Gunther here."

"Her? Phoebe Gunther?"

"Yes."

"That's dangerous. Isn't it too risky to trust me with her?"

"Yes. But I want to see her."

"Okay, it's on you."

16.

Two hours and more of back-breaking drudgery. Ten whole cylinders. Three carbons. Not only that, it was new to me and I had to adjust the speed about twenty times before I got the knack of it. When I finally got it finished and the sheets collated, I gave the original to Wolfe, who was back in the office by that time, placed the first two carbons in the safe, and folded the third carbon and stuck it in my pocket. Then there were the dozen letters to be typed and envelopes for same. As Wolfe signed them he folded and inserted them, and even sealed the envelopes. Sometimes he has bursts of feverish energy that are uncontrollable. By that time it was the dinner hour, but I decided not to dawdle through a meal in the dining room with Wolfe and made a quickie of it in the kitchen.

I had phoned the Homicide Squad office to make sure that Cramer would be on hand, to avoid having to deal with Lieutenant Rowcliffe, whose murder I hoped to help investigate some day, and had also called Phoebe Gunther's apartment to make a date but got no answer. Getting the car from the garage, I went first to Eighth Avenue to drop the letters in the post office and then headed south for Twentieth Street.

After I had been in with Cramer ten minutes he said, "This sounds like something. I'll be damned."

After another twenty minutes he said, "This sounds like something. I'll be damned."

That, of course, showed clear as day where he stood—up to his hips in a swamp. If he had been anywhere near dry ground, or even in sight of some, he would have waved his prerogative in front of my nose and cussed Wolfe and me up one side and down the other for withholding evidence for nine hours and fourteen minutes and so forth, including threats, growls, and warnings. Instead of which, at one point it looked as if he might abandon all restraint and thank me. Obviously he was desperate.

When I left Cramer I still had the carbon of the transcription in my pocket, because it was not intended for him. If I was to take Phoebe Gunther to Wolfe it was desirable that I get her before Cramer did, and it seemed likely that he would want to know exactly what was on those cylinders before he started a roundup. So I had kept it sketchy and hadn't told him that a transcription had been made.

Also I wasted no time getting to Fifty-fifth Street.

The doorman phoned up, gave me another look of surprise when he turned to tell me I would be received, and called an okay to the elevator. Up at Nine H, Phoebe opened the door and allowed me to enter. I put my coat and hat on a chair and followed her into the room, and there was Alger Kates over in the corner where the light was dim.

I will not deny that I am often forthright, but I would put up an argument if anyone called me crude. Yet, at sight of Kates there again, I said what I said. I suppose it could be interpreted different ways. I do not concede that Phoebe Gunther had me fidgeting on a string, but the fact remains that I stared at Alger Kates and demanded:

"Do you live here?"

He stared back and replied, "If it's any of your business, yes, I do."

"Sit down, Mr. Goodwin." Phoebe possibly smiled. She got against the cushions on the couch. "I'll straighten it out. Mr. Kates does live here, when he's in New York. His wife keeps this apartment because she can't stand Washington. Right now she's in Florida. I couldn't get a hotel room, so Mr. Kates is staying with friends on Eleventh Street and letting me sleep here. Does that clear me? And him?"

Naturally I felt foolish. "I'll take it up," I said, "with the Housing Administration and see what I can do. Meanwhile I may be in a hurry, depending on how urgent Inspector Cramer feels. When I phoned you about an hour ago there was no answer."

She reached for a cigarette. "Why, do I need clearance on that too? I was out for a bite to eat."

"Has Cramer's office called since you returned?"

"No." She was frowning. "Does he want me? What for?"

"He either wants you now or he soon will." It was in the line of duty to keep my eyes fastened to her, to get her reaction. "I just took him that case of cylinders that you left on a window sill Tuesday evening."

I do not believe there was any menace in my tone. I don't know where it would have come from, as I did not at that time regard myself as a menace to Miss Gunther. But Alger Kates suddenly stood up, as if I had brandished a monkey wrench at her. He immediately sat down again. She kept her seat, but stopped her cigarette abruptly on its way to her lips, and the muscles of her neck stiffened.

"That case? With the cylinders in it?"

"Yes, ma'am."

"Did you—what's on them?"

"Well, that's a long story—"

"Where did you find it?"

"That's another long story. We've got to step on it, because Cramer has it now, and he may send for you any minute, or come to see you, or he may wait until he has listened to the cylinders. Anyhow, Mr. Wolfe wants to see you first, and since it was me—"

"Then you don't know what's on them?"

Kates had left his dim corner and moved across to the end of the couch, and was standing there in an attitude of readiness to repel the enemy. I ignored him and told her:

"Sure, I know. So does Mr. Wolfe. We got a machine and ran them off. They're interesting but not helpful. Their outstanding feature is that they weren't dictated on Tuesday, but before that—some of them a week or more. I'll tell—"

"But that's impossible!"

"Nope. Possible and true. I'll—"

"How do you know?"

"Dates and things. Absolutely." I stood up. "I'm getting restless. As I say, Mr. Wolfe wants to see you first. With Cramer there's no telling, especially when he's hanging on by his fingernails, so let's go. Kates can come along to protect you if you want him to. I've got a transcription of the cylinders in my pocket and you can look at it on the way, and I'll tell—"

A bell rang. Having, though from the outside, heard it ring twice previously, I knew what it was.

I thought goddam it. I asked her in a whisper, "You expecting anybody?"

She shook her head, and the look in her eyes, straight at mine, said plainly that I could name the tune. But of course it was hopeless. Whoever had got by the doorman had also got information. Even so, there's nothing like trying, so I put a finger to my lips and stood there looking at them—at least I gave Kates a glance. His expression said belligerently, I'm not doing this for *you,* mister. We had held the tableau maybe ten seconds when a voice I knew well, the voice of Sergeant Purley Stebbins, came loud and irritated through the door:

"Come on, Goodwin, what the hell!"

I marched across and opened up. He came in past me rudely, took off his hat, and began to try to pretend he was a gentleman.

"Good afternoon, Miss Gunther. Good afternoon, Mr. Kates." He looked at her. "Inspector Cramer would be much obliged if you'd let me drive you down to his office. He's got some things there he wants you to look at. He told me to tell you they're Stenophone cylinders."

I was at his side. "You come right to the point, don't you, Purley, huh?"

"Oh," he said, pivoting his big fine empty head, "you still here? I supposed you was gone. The Inspector will be glad to know I ran into you."

"Nuts." I dropped him. "Of course you know, Miss Gunther, that you may do as you please. Some people think that when a city employee comes to take them somewhere they have to go. That's a fallacy, unless he has a document, which he hasn't."

"Is that true?" she asked me.

"Yes. That's true."

She had stood up when Purley entered. Now she moved across right to me, facing me, and stood looking up to meet my eyes. It wasn't much of a slant, because her eyes were only about five inches below mine, and therefore it wasn't a strain for either of us.

"You know," she said, "you have a way of suggesting things that appeal to me. With all I know about cops and their attitude toward people with power and position and money, and with the little I know about you, even if your boss has been hired by the NIA, I almost think I would let you hold my purse if I had to fix my garter. So you decide for me. I'll go with you to see Mr. Wolfe, or I'll go with this oversize sergeant, whichever you say."

Whereupon I made a mistake. It isn't so much that I regret it because it was a mistake, since I believe in having my share of everything on my way through life, including mistakes. The trouble was, as I now admit, that I did it not for my sake, or for Wolfe's, or for the good of the job, but for her. I would have loved to escort her down to my car with Purley traipsing along behind growling. Wolfe liked nothing better than to rile Cramer. But I knew if I took her to Wolfe's house Purley would camp outside, and after Wolfe finished with her she would either go on downtown for a night of it, or she would refuse to go, and she would certainly never hear the last of that. So I made the mistake because I thought Miss Gunther should have some sleep. Since she had told me herself that the tireder she got the better she looked, and there I was looking at her, it was evident that she was about all in.

So I said, "I deeply appreciate your confidence, which I deserve. You hold onto the purse while I fix the garter. For the present, I hate to say it, but it would be better to accept Cramer's invitation. I'll be seeing you."

Twenty minutes later I walked into the office and told Wolfe:

"Purley Stebbins arrived at Miss Gunther's before I could get her away, and she likes him better than she does me. She is now down at Twentieth Street."

So not only had I made a mistake, but also I was lying to the boss.

17.

MONDAY would fill a book if I let it, and so would any other day, I suppose, if you put it all in.

First thing in the morning Wolfe provided evidence of how we were doing, or rather not doing, by having Saul Panzer and Bill Gore sent up to his room during the breakfast hour for private instructions. That was one of his established dodges for trying to keep me from needling him. The theory was that if I contributed any remarks about inertia or age beginning to tell or anything like that, he could shut me up by intimating that he was working like a demon supervising Saul and Bill, and they were gathering in the sheaves. Also that it wouldn't be safe to let me in on the secret because I couldn't control my face. One reason that got my goat was that I knew that he knew it wasn't true.

The sheaves they had so far delivered had not relieved the famine. The armful of words, typed, printed and mimeographed, that Bill Gore had brought in from the NIA would have kept the *Time* and *Life* research staff out of mischief for a week, and that was about all it was good for. Saul Panzer's report on his week end at the Waldorf was what you would expect, no man whose initials were not A.G. could have done better, but all it added up to was that no hair of a murderer's head was to be found on the premises. What Wolfe was continuing to shell out fifty bucks a day for was, as I say, presumably none of my business.

Public Relations had tottered to its feet again, taken a deep breath, and let out a battle cry. There was a full page ad in the *Times,* signed by the National Industrial Association, warning us that the Bureau of Price Regulation, after depriving us of our shirts and pants, was all set to peel off our hides. While there was no mention of homicide, the implication was that since it was still necessary for the NIA to save the country from the vicious deep-laid plots of the BPR, it was silly to imagine that it had any hand in the bumping off of Cheney

Boone. As strategy, the hitch in it was that it would work only with those who already agreed with the NIA regarding who or what had got the shirts and pants.

One of my Monday problems was to get my outgoing phone calls made, on account of so many coming in the other direction. I started bright and early after Phoebe Gunther and never did get her. First, from the Fifty-fifth Street apartment, I got no answer. At nine-thirty I tried the BPR office and was told she hadn't arrived, and no one seemed to know whether she was expected. At ten-thirty I was informed that she was there, but was in with Mr. Dexter and would I call later. Twice later, before noon, she was still with Mr. Dexter. At twelve-thirty she had gone to lunch; my message for her to call me had been given to her. At one-thirty she wasn't back yet. At two o'clock the word was that she wouldn't be back, and no one that I got to knew where she was. That may all sound as if I am a push-over for a runaround, but I had two strikes on me all the way. Apparently there was nobody at the BPR, from switchboard girls to the Regional Director, who didn't know that Nero Wolfe, as Alger Kates put it, was in the pay of NIA, and they reacted accordingly. When I made an attempt to get connected with Dorothy Unger, the stenographer who had phoned Don O'Neill Saturday evening to ask him to mail her the parcel check which she had enclosed in his envelope by mistake, I couldn't even find anyone who would even admit he had ever heard of her.

What I got for my money on phone calls that day was enough to send Tel & Tel to a new low. On incoming calls the score was no better. In addition to the usual routine on a big case, like newspaper boys wanting a ringside seat in case Nero Wolfe was winding up for another fast one, there were all kinds of client trouble on account of the letters Wolfe had sent about finding the cylinders. The ad in the *Times* may have indicated that the NIA was a united front, but the phone calls didn't. Each one had a different slant. Winterhoff's line was that the assumption in the letter that the manner of finding the cylinders vindicated Miss Gunther was unjustified; that on the contrary it reinforced the suspicion that Miss Gunther was lying about it, since the parcel check had been mailed to Don O'Neill in a BPR envelope. Breslow, of course, was angry, so much so that he phoned twice, once in the morning and once in the afternoon. What had him sore this time was that we had spread the news about the cylinders. In the interests of justice we should have kept it to ourselves and the cops. He accused us of trying to make an impression on the Executive Committee, of trying to show that we were earning our money, and that was a hell of a note; we should have only two things in mind: the apprehension of the criminal and the proof of his guilt.

Even the Erskine family was divided. Frank Thomas Erskine, the father, had no complaint or criticism. He simply wanted something: namely, the full text of what was on the cylinders. He didn't get indignant but he was utterly astonished. To him the situation was plain. Wolfe was doing a paid job for the NIA, and any information he got in the performance of that job was the property of the NIA, and any attempt to exclude them from possession of their property was felonious, malevolent, and naughty. He insisted as long as he thought there was any chance, and then quit without any indications of hard feelings.

The son, Ed, was the shortest and funniest. All the others had demanded to talk to Wolfe, not just me, but he said it didn't matter, I would do fine, all he wanted was to ask a question. I said shoot, and he asked this, "How good is the evidence that O'Neill got the parcel check the way he says he did, in the mail?" I said that all we had, besides a look at the envelope, was O'Neill's say-so, but that of course the police were checking it and he'd better ask them. He said much obliged and hung up.

All day I kept expecting a call from Don O'Neill, but there wasn't a peep out of him.

The general impression I got was that the Executive Committee had better call a meeting and decide on policy.

The day went, and dusk came, and I turned on lights. Just before dinner I tried Fifty-fifth Street, but no Phoebe Gunther. The meal took even longer than usual, which is to be expected when Wolfe is completely at a loss. He uses up energy keeping thoughts out and trying to keep me quiet, and that makes him eat more. After dinner, back in the office, I tried Fifty-fifth Street once more, with the same result. I was stretched out on the couch, trying to work out an attack that would make Wolfe explode into some kind of action, when the bell rang and I went to the front door and swung it wide open without a preliminary peek through the glass. As far as I was concerned anybody at all would have been welcome, even Breslow, just for a friendly chat.

Two men stepped in. I told them to hang up their things and went to the office door and announced:

"Inspector Cramer and Mr. Solomon Dexter."

Wolfe sighed and muttered, "Bring them in."

18.

Solomon Dexter was a blurter. I suppose, as Acting Director of BPR, he had enough to make him blurt, what with this and that, including things like Congress in an election year and the NIA ad in the morning *Times,* not to mention the unsolved murder of his predecessor, but still Wolfe does not like blurters. So he listened with a frown when, after brief greetings and with no preamble, Dexter blurted:

"I don't understand it at all! I've checked on you with the FBI and the Army, and they give you a clean bill and speak of you very highly! And here you are tied up with the dirtiest bunch of liars and cutthroats in existence! What the hell is the idea?"

"Your nerves are on edge," Wolfe said.

He blurted some more. "What have my nerves got to do with it? The blackest crime in the history of this country, with that unscrupulous gang behind it, and any man, any man whatever, who ties himself up—"

"Please!" Wolfe snapped. "Don't shout at me like that. You're excited. Justifiably excited perhaps, but Mr. Cramer shouldn't have brought you in here until you had cooled off." His eyes moved. "What does he want, Mr. Cramer? Does he want something?"

"Yeah," Cramer growled. "He thinks you fixed that stunt about the cylinders. So it would look as if the BPR had them all the time and tried to plant them on the NIA."

"Pfui. Do you think so too?"

"I do not. You would have done a better job of it."

Wolfe's eyes moved again. "If that's what you want, Mr. Dexter, to ask me if I arranged some flummery about those cylinders, the answer is I didn't. Anything else?"

Dexter had taken a handkerchief from his pocket and was mopping his face. I hadn't noticed any moisture on him, and it was cool out, and we keep the room at seventy, but apparently he felt that there was something to mop. That was probably the lumberjack in him. He dropped his hand to his thigh, clutching the handkerchief, and looked at Wolfe as if he were trying to remember the next line of the script.

"There is no one," he said, "by the name of Dorothy Unger employed by the BPR, either in New York or Washington."

"Good heavens." Wolfe was exasperated. "Of course there isn't."

"What do you mean of course there isn't?"

"I mean it's obvious there wouldn't be. Whoever contrived that hocus-pocus about the parcel check, whether Mr. O'Neill himself or someone else, certainly Dorothy Unger had to be invented."

"You ought to know," Dexter asserted savagely.

"Nonsense." Wolfe moved a finger to brush him away. "Mr. Dexter. If you're going to sit there and boil with suspicion you might as well leave. You accuse me of being 'tied up' with miscreants. I am 'tied up' with no one. I have engaged to do a specific job, find a murderer and get enough evidence to convict him. If you have any—"

"How far have you got?" Cramer interrupted.

"Well." Wolfe smirked. He is most intolerable when he smirks. "Further than you, or you wouldn't be here."

"Yeah," Cramer said sarcastically. "Here the other evening, I didn't quite understand why you didn't pick him out and let me take him."

"Neither did I," Wolfe agreed. "For one moment I thought I might, when one of them said something extraordinary, but I was unable—"

"Who said what?"

Wolfe shook his head. "I'm having it looked into." His tone implied that the 82nd Airborne was at it from coast to coast. He shifted to one of mild reproach. "You broke it up and chased them out. If you had acted like an adult investigator instead of an ill-tempered child I might have got somewhere."

"Oh, sure. I bitched it for you. I'd do anything to square it, anything you say. Why don't you ask me to get them all in here again, right now?"

"An excellent idea." Wolfe nearly sat up straight, he was so overcome with enthusiasm. "Excellent. I do ask it. Use Mr. Goodwin's phone."

"By God!" Cramer stared. "You thought I meant it?"

"*I* mean it," Wolfe asserted. "You wouldn't be here if you weren't desperate. You wouldn't be desperate if you could think of any more questions to ask anyone. That's what you came to me for, to get ideas for more questions. Get those people here, and I'll see what I can do."

"Who the hell does this man think he is?" Dexter demanded of Cramer.

Cramer, scowling at Wolfe, didn't reply. After some seconds he arose and, without any alteration in the scowl, came to my desk. By the time he arrived I had lifted the receiver and started to dial Watkins 9-8242. He took it, sat on the corner of the desk, and went on scowling.

"Horowitz? Inspector Cramer, talking from Nero Wolfe's office. Give me Lieutenant Rowcliffe. George? No, what do you expect, I just got here. Anything from on high? Yeah. Yeah? File it under C for crap. No. You've got a list of the people who were here at Wolfe's Friday evening. Get some help on the phones and call all of them and tell them to come to Wolfe's office immediately. I know that, but *tell* them. You'd better include Phoebe Gunther. Wait a minute."

He turned to Wolfe. "Anyone else?" Wolfe shook his head and Cramer resumed:

"That's all. Send Stebbins here right away. Wherever they are, find them and get them here. Send men out if you have to. Yeah, I know, all right, they raise hell, what's the difference how I lose my job if I lose it? Wolfe says I'm desperate, and you know Wolfe, he reads faces. Step on it."

Cramer went back to the red leather chair, sat, pulled out a cigar and sank his teeth in it, and rasped, "There. I never thought I'd come to this."

"Frankly," Wolfe muttered, "I was surprised to see you. With what Mr. Goodwin and I furnished you yesterday I would have guessed you were making headway."

"Sure," Cramer chewed the cigar. "Headway in the thickest damn fog I ever saw. That was a big help, what you and Goodwin furnished. In the first place—"

"Excuse me," Dexter put in. He stood up. "I have some phone calls to make."

"If they're private," I told him, "there's a phone upstairs you can use."

"No, thanks." He looked at me impolitely. "I'll go and find a booth." He started out, halted to say over his shoulder that he would be back in half an hour, and went. I moseyed to the hall to see that he didn't stumble on the sill, and after the door had closed behind him returned to the office. Cramer was talking:

". . . and we're worse off than we were before. Zeros all the way across. If you care for any details, take your pick."

Wolfe grunted. "The photograph and car license mailed to Mrs. Boone. The envelope. Will you have some beer?"

"Yes, I will. Fingerprints, all the routine, nothing. Mailed midtown Friday eight P.M. How would you like to check sales of envelopes in the five-and-dimes?"

"Archie might try it." It was a sign we were all good friends when Wolfe, speaking to Cramer, called me Archie. Usually it was Mr. Goodwin. "What about those cylinders?"

"They were dictated by Boone on March 19th and typed by Miss Gunther on the 20th. The carbons are in Washington and the FBI has checked them. Miss Gunther can't understand it, except on the assumption that Boone picked up the wrong case when he left his office Tuesday afternoon, and she says he didn't often make mistakes like that. But if that was it the case containing the cylinders he dictated Tuesday afternoon ought to be still in his office in Washington, and it isn't. No sign of it. There's one other possibility. We've asked everyone concerned not to leave the city, but on Thursday the BPR asked permission for Miss Gunther to go to Washington on urgent business, and we let her. She flew down and back. She had a suitcase with her."

Wolfe shuddered. The idea of people getting on airplanes voluntarily was too much for him. He flashed a glance at Cramer. "I see you have eliminated nothing. Was Miss Gunther alone on her trip?"

"She went down alone. Dexter and two other BPR men came back with her."

"She has no difficulty explaining her movements?"

"She has no difficulty explaining anything. That young woman has no difficulty explaining period."

Wolfe nodded. "I believe Archie agrees with you." The beer had arrived, escorted by Fritz, and he was pouring. "I suppose you've had a talk with Mr. O'Neill."

"A talk?" Cramer raised his hands. one of them holding a glass of beer. "Saint Agnes! Have I had a talk with that bird!"

"Yes, he talks. As Archie told you, he was curious about what was on those cylinders."

"He still is." Cramer had half emptied his glass and hung onto it. "The damn fool thought he could keep that envelope. He wanted to have a private dick, not you, investigate it, so he said." He drank again. "Now there's an example of what this case is like. Would you want a better lead than an envelope like that? BPR stock, special delivery, one stamp canceled and the others not, typewritten address? Shall I tell you in detail what we've done, including trying a thousand typewriters?"

"I think not."

"I think not too. It would only take all night to tell you. The goddam post office says it's too bad they can't help us, but with all the new girls they've got, stamps canceled, stamps not canceled, you never can tell." Cramer emptied the bottle into the glass. "You heard that crack I made to Rowcliffe about my losing my job."

"That?" Wolfe waved it away.

"Yeah, I know," Cramer agreed, "I've made it before. It's a habit. All inspectors tell their wives every evening that they'll probably be captains tomorrow. But this time I don't know. From the standpoint of a Homicide Squad inspector, an atom bomb would be a baby firecracker compared to this damn thing. The Commissioner has got St. Vitus's Dance. The D.A. is trying to pretend his turn doesn't come until it's time to panel a jury. The Mayor is having nightmares, and he must have got it in a dream that if there wasn't any Homicide Squad there wouldn't be any murders, at least not any involving big-time citizens. So it's all my fault. I mustn't get tough with refined people who have got to the point where they employ tax experts to make sure they're not cheating the government. On the other hand, I must realize that public sentiment absolutely demands that the murderer of Cheney Boone shall not go unpunished. It's six days since it happened, and here by God I sit beefing to you."

He drank his glass empty, put it down, and used the back of his hand for a napkin. "That's the situation, my fat friend, as Charlie McCarthy said to Herbert Hoover. Look what I'm doing, letting you take the wheel is what it amounts to, at least long enough for you to run me in a ditch if you happen to need to. I know damn well that no client of yours has ever been convicted of murder, and in this case your clients—"

"No man is my client," Wolfe interposed. "My client is an association. An association can't commit murder."

"Maybe not. Even so, I know how you work. If you thought it was necessary, in the interest of your client—I guess here he comes or here it comes."

The doorbell had rung. I went to answer it, and found that Cramer's guess was right. This first arrival was a piece of our client, in the person of Hattie Harding. She seemed out of breath. There in the hall she gripped my arm and wanted to know:

"What is it? Have they—what is it?"

I used the hand of my other arm to pat her shoulder. "No, no, calm down. You're all tense. We've decided to have these affairs twice a week, that's all."

I took her to the office and put her to helping me with chairs.

From then on they dribbled in, one by one. Purley Stebbins arrived and apologized to his boss for not making it quicker, and took him aside to explain something. G. G. Spero of the FBI was third and Mrs. Boone fourth. Along about the middle Solomon Dexter returned, and finding the red leather chair unoccupied at the moment, copped it for himself. The Erskine family came separately, a quarter of an hour apart, and so did Breslow and Winterhoff. On the whole, as I let them in, they returned my greeting as a fellow member of the human race, one world or none, but there were two exceptions. Don O'Neill looked straight through me and conveyed the impression that if I touched his coat it would have to be sent to the cleaners, so I let him put it on the rack himself. Alger Kates acted as if I was paid to do the job, so no embraces were called for. Nina Boone, who came late, smiled at me. I didn't imagine it; she smiled right at me. To repay her, I saw to it that she got the same position she had had before, the chair next to mine.

I had to hand it to the Police Department as inviters. It was ten-forty, just an hour and ten minutes since Cramer had phoned Rowcliffe to get up a party. I stood and looked them over, checking off, and then turned to Wolfe and told him:

"It's the same as last time. Miss Gunther just doesn't like crowds. They're all here except her."

Wolfe moved his eyes over the assemblage, slowly from right to left and back again, like a man trying to make up his mind which shirt to buy. They were all seated, divided into two camps as before, except that Winterhoff and Erskine the father were standing over by the globe talking in undertones. From the standpoint of gaiety the party was a dud before it ever started. One second there would be a buzz of conversation, and the next second dead silence; then that would get on someone's nerves and the buzz would start again. A photographer could have taken a shot of that collection of faces and called it I Wonder Who's Kissing Her Now.

Cramer came to my desk and used the phone and then told Wolfe, leaning over to him, "They got Miss Gunther at her apartment over an hour ago, and she said she'd come immediately."

Wolfe shrugged. "We won't wait. Go ahead."

Cramer turned to face the guests, cleared his throat, and raised his voice:

"Ladies and gentlemen!" There was instant silence. "I want you to understand why you were asked to come here, and exactly what's going on. I suppose you read the papers. According to the papers, at least some of them, the police are finding this case too hot to handle on account of the people involved, and they're laying down on the job. I think every single person here knows how much truth there is in that. I guess all of you feel, or nearly all of you, that you're being pestered and persecuted on account of something that you had nothing to do with. The newspapers have their angle, and you have yours. I suppose it was an inconvenience to all of you to come here this evening, but you've got to face it that there's no way out of it, and you've got to blame that inconvenience not on the police or anybody else except one person, the person who killed Cheney Boone. I'm not saying that person is in this room. I admit I don't know. He may be a thousand miles from here—"

"Is that," Breslow barked, "what you got us here to listen to? We've heard all that before!"

"Yeah, I know you have." Cramer was trying not to sound sour. "We didn't get you here to listen to me. I am now turning this over to Mr. Wolfe, and he will proceed, after I say two things. First, you got the request to come here from my office, but from here on it is not official. I am responsible for getting you here and that's all. As far as I'm concerned you can all get up and go if you feel like it. Second, some of you may feel that this is improper because Mr. Wolfe has been engaged to work on this case by the National Industrial Association. That may be so. All I can say is, if you feel that way you can stay here and keep that in mind, or you can leave. Suit yourselves."

He looked around. Nobody moved or spoke. Cramer waited ten seconds and then turned and nodded at Wolfe.

Wolfe heaved a deep high and opened up with a barely audible murmur:

"One thing Mr. Cramer mentioned, the inconvenience you people are being forced to endure, requires a little comment. I ask your forbearance while I make it. It is only by that kind of sacrifice on the part of persons, sometimes many persons, who are themselves wholly blameless—"

I hated to disturb his flow, because I knew from long experience that at last he was really working. He had resolved to get something out of that bunch if he had to keep them there all night. But there was no help for it, on account of the expression on Fritz's face. A movement out in the hall had caught my eye, and Fritz was standing there, four feet back from the door to the office, which was standing open, staring wide-eyed at me. When he saw I was looking at him he beckoned to me to come, and the thought popped into my mind that, with guests present and Wolfe making an oration, that was precisely how Fritz would act if the house was on fire. The whole throng was between him and me, and I circled around behind them for my exit. Wolfe kept on talking. As soon as I made the hall I closed the door behind me and asked Fritz:

"Something biting you?"

"It's—it's—" He stopped and set his teeth on his lip. Wolfe had been trying to train Fritz for twenty years not to get excited. He tried again: "Come and I'll show you."

He dived for the kitchen and I followed, thinking it was some culinary calamity that he couldn't bear up under alone, but he went to the door to the back stairs, the steps that led down to what we called the basement, though it was only three feet below the street level. Fritz slept down there in the room that faced the street. There was an exit through a little hall to the front; first a heavy door out to a tiny vestibule which was underneath the stoop, and then an iron gate, a grill, leading to a paved areaway from which five steps mounted to the sidewalk. It was in the tiny vestibule that Fritz stopped and I bumped into him.

He pointed down. "Look." He put his hand on the gate and gave it a little shake. "I came to see if the gate was locked, the way I always do."

There was an object huddled on the concrete of the areaway, up against the gate, so that the gate couldn't be opened without pushing the object aside. I squatted to peer. The light there was dim, since the nearest street lamp was on the other side of the stoop, thirty paces away, but I could see well enough to tell what the object was, though not for certain who it was.

"What the hell did you bring me here for?" I demanded, pushing past Fritz to re-enter the basement. "Come with me."

He was at my heels as I mounted the stairs. In the kitchen I detoured to jerk open a drawer and get a flashlight, and then went down the main hall to the front door, out to the stoop and down to the sidewalk, and down the five steps to the areaway. There, on the same side of the gate as the object, I squatted again and switched on the flashlight. Fritz was beside me, bending over.

"Shall I—" His voice was shaking and he had to start again. "Shall I hold the light?"

I told him gruffly, "Shut up, goddam it."

After half a minute I straightened up, told him, "You stay right here," and headed for the stoop. Fritz had pulled the front door shut, and when I found myself fumbling to get the key in the hole I stood erect to take a deep breath and that stopped the fumbling. I went down the hall to the kitchen, to the phone there, and dialed the number of Dr. Vollmer, who lived down the street only half a block away. There were six buzzes before he answered.

"Doc? Archie Goodwin. Got your clothes on? Good. Get here as fast as you can. There's a woman lying in our areaway, by the gate to the basement, been hit on the head, and I think she's dead. There'll be cops on it, so don't shift her more than you have to. Right now? Okay."

I took another breath, filling my chest, then took Fritz's pad and pencil and wrote:

Phoebe Gunther is in our areaway dead. Hit on the head. Have phoned Vollmer.

I tore off the sheet and went to the office. I suppose I had been gone six minutes, not more, and Wolfe was still doing a monologue, with thirteen pairs of eyes riveted on him. I sidled around to the right, got to his desk, and handed him the note. He got it at a glance, gave it a longer glance, flashed one at me, and spoke without any perceptible change in tone or manner:

"Mr. Cramer. If you please. Mr. Goodwin has a message for you and Mr. Stebbins. Will you go with him to the hall?"

Cramer and Stebbins got up. As we went out Wolfe's voice was resuming behind us:

"Now the question that confronts us is whether it is credible, under the circumstances as we know them . . ."

19.

THIRTY minutes past midnight was about the peak. At that moment I was alone in my room, two flights up, sitting in the chair by the window, drinking a glass of milk, or at least holding one in my hand. I do not ordinarily hunt for a cave in the middle of the biggest excitement and the most intense action, but this seemed to hit me in a new spot or something, and anyhow there I was, trying to arrange my mind. Or maybe my feelings. All I knew was that something inside of me needed a little arranging. I had just completed a tour of the battlefield, and at that hour the disposition of forces was as follows:

Fritz was in the kitchen making sandwiches and coffee, and Mrs. Boone was there helping him.

Seven of the invited guests were scattered around the front room, with two homicide dicks keeping them company. They were not telling funny stories, not even Ed Erskine and Nina Boone, who were on the same sofa.

Lieutenant Rowcliffe and an underling with a notebook were in the spare bedroom, on the same floor as mine, having a conversation with Hattie Harding, the Public Relations Queen.

Inspector Cramer, Sergeant Stebbins, and a couple of others were in the dining room firing questions at Alger Kates.

The four-star brass was in the office. Wolfe was seated behind his desk, the Police Commissioner was likewise at my desk, the District Attorney was in the red leather chair, and Travis and Spero of the FBI made a circle of it. That was where the high strategy would come from, if and when any came.

Another dick was in the kitchen, presumably to see that Mrs. Boone didn't jump out a window and Fritz didn't dust arsenic on the sandwiches. Others were in the halls, in the basement, all over; and still others kept coming and going from outdoors, reporting to, or getting orders from, Cramer or the Commissioner or the District Attorney.

Newspapermen had at one time infiltrated behind the lines, but they were now on the other side of the threshold. Out there the floodlights hadn't been removed, and some miscellaneous city employees were still poking around, but most of the scientists, including the photographers, had departed. In spite of that the crowd, as I could see from the window near which my chair was placed, was bigger than ever. The house was only a five-minute taxi ride or a fifteen-minute walk from Times Square, and the news of a spectacular break in the Boone case had got to the theater crowds. The little party Wolfe had asked Cramer to arrange had developed into more than he had bargained for.

A piece of 1½-inch iron pipe, sixteen inches long, had been found lying on the concrete paving of the areaway. Phoebe Gunther had been hit on the head with it four times. Dr. Vollmer had certified her dead on arrival. She had also received bruises in falling, one on her cheek and mouth, presumably from the stoop, where she had been struck, to the areaway. The scientists had got that far before they removed the body.

I had been sitting in my room twenty minutes when I noticed that I hadn't drunk any milk, but I hadn't spilled any from the glass.

20.

My intention was to go back downstairs and re-enter the turmoil when the microscope came. It was expected by some that the microscope would do the job, and it seemed to me quite likely.

I had myself been rinsed out, by Wolfe and Cramer working as a team, which alone made the case unique. But the circumstances made me a key man. The working assumption was that Phoebe had come and mounted the stoop, and that the murderer had either come with her, or joined her near or on the stoop, and had struck her before she had pushed the bell button, stunning her and knocking her off the stoop into the areaway. He had then run down into the areaway and hit her three times more to make sure she was finished, and shoved the body up against the gate, where it could not be seen by anyone on the stoop without leaning over and stretching your neck, and wasn't likely to be seen from the sidewalk on account of the dimness of the light. Then, of course, the murderer might have gone home and to bed, but the assumption was that he had remounted the stoop and pushed the button, and I had let him in and taken his hat and coat.

That put me within ten feet of them, and maybe less, at the moment it happened, and if by chance I had pulled the curtain on the glass panel aside at that moment I would have seen it. It also had me greeting the murderer within a few seconds after he had finished, and, as I admitted to Wolfe and Cramer, I had observed each arriving face with both eyes to discover how they were getting along under the strain. That was another reason I had gone up to my room, to look back on those faces. It didn't seem possible that I couldn't pick the one, or at least the two or three most probable ones, whose owner had just a minute previously been smashing Phoebe's skull with an iron pipe. Well, I couldn't. They had all been the opposite of carefree, showing it one way or another, and so what? Wolfe had sighed at me, and Cramer had growled like a frustrated lion, but that was the best I could do.

Naturally I had been asked to make up a list showing the order of arrivals and the approximate intervals between, and had been glad to oblige. I hadn't punched a time clock for them, but I was willing to certify my list as pretty accurate. They had all come singly. The idea was that if any two of them had arrived close together, say within two minutes or less of each other, the one that entered the house first could be marked as improbable. But not the one that came in second, because the murderer, having finished, and hearing footsteps or a taxi approaching, could have flattened himself against the gate in that dark corner, waited until the arriver had mounted the stoop and been admitted. and then immediately ascended the stoop himself to ring the bell. Anyhow, such close calculation wasn't required, since, as my memory had it, none of the intervals had been less than three minutes.

Of course the position on the list meant nothing. As far as opportunity was concerned, there was no difference between Hattie Harding, who came first, and Nina Boone, who came last.

All the guests had been questioned at least once, each separately, and it was probable that repeat performances would go on all night if the microscope didn't live up to expectations. Since they had all already been put through it, over and over, about the Boone murder, the askers had hard going. The questions had to be about what had happened there that evening, and what was there to ask? There was no such thing as an alibi. Each one had been on the stoop alone between nine-fifty and ten-forty, and during that period Phoebe Gunther had arrived and been killed. About all you could ask anybody was this, "Did you ring the bell as soon as you mounted the stoop? Did you kill Phoebe Gunther first?" If he said Phoebe Gunther wasn't there, and he pushed the button and was admitted by Mr. Goodwin, what did you ask next? Naturally you wanted to know whether he came by car or taxi, or on foot from a bus or subway, and where did that get you?

Very neat management, I told myself, sitting by the window in my room. Fully as neat as any I remembered. Very neat, the dirty deadly bastard.

I have said that the assumption was that the murderer had remounted the stoop and entered the house, but perhaps I should have said one of the assumptions. The NIA had another one, originated by Winterhoff, which had been made a part of the record. In the questioning marathon Winterhoff had come toward the end. His story had three main ingredients:

1. He (Winterhoff, the Man of Distinction) always had shoe soles made of a composition which was almost as quiet as rubber, and therefore made little noise when he walked.

2. He disapproved of tossing trash, including cigarette butts, in the street, and never did so himself.

3. He lived on East End Avenue. His wife and daughters were using the car and chauffeur that evening. He never used taxis if he could help it, because of the revolutionary attitude of the drivers during the present shortage of cabs. So when the phone call had come requesting his presence at Wolfe's office, he had taken a Second Avenue bus down to Thirty-fifth Street, and walked crosstown.

Well. Approaching Wolfe's house from the east, on his silent soles, he had stopped about eighty feet short of his destination because he was stuck with a cigarette butt and noticed an ashcan standing inside the railing of an areaway. He went down the steps to the can and killed the butt therein, and, ascending the steps, was barely back to the sidewalk when he saw a man dart out from behind a stoop, out of an areaway, and dash off in the other direction, toward the river. He had gone on to Wolfe's house, and had noted that it was that areaway, probably, that the man had darted from, but he had not gone so far as to lean over the stoop's low parapet to peer into the areaway. The best he could do on the darting and dashing man was that he had worn dark clothes and had been neither a giant nor a midget.

And by gosh, there had been corroboration. Of the thousand more or less dicks who had been dispatched on errands, two had been sent up the street to check. In half an hour they had returned and reported that there was an ashcan in an areaway exactly twenty-four paces east of Wolfe's stoop. Not only that, there was a cigarette butt on top of the ashes, and its condition, and certain telltale streaks on the inside of the can, about one inch below its rim, made it probable that the butt had been killed by rubbing it against the inside of the can. Not only *that*, they had the butt with them.

Winterhoff had not lied. He had stopped to kill a butt in an ashcan, and he was a good judge of distances. Unfortunately, it was impossible to corroborate the part about the darting and dashing man because he had disappeared during the two hours that had elapsed.

How much Wolfe or Cramer had bought of it, I didn't know. I wasn't even sure how well I liked it, but I had been below normal since I had flashed the light on Phoebe Gunther's face.

Cramer, hearing it from Rowcliffe, who had questioned Winterhoff, had merely grunted, but that had apparently been because at the moment he had his mind on something else. Some scientist, I never knew which one, had just made the suggestion about the microscope. Cramer lost no time on that. He gave orders that Erskine and Dexter, who were elsewhere being questioned, should be returned immediately to the front room, and had then gone there himself, accompanied by Purley and me, stood facing the assemblage and got their attention, which took no effort at all, and had begun a speech:

"Please listen to this closely so you'll know what I'm asking. The piece of—"

Breslow blurted, "This is outrageous! We've all answered questions! We've let ourselves be searched! We've told everything we know! We—"

Cramer told a dick in a loud and hard voice, "Go and stand by him and if he doesn't keep his trap shut, shut it."

The dick moved. Breslow stopped blurting. Cramer said: "I've had enough injured innocence for one night." He was as sore and savage as I had ever seen him. "For six days I've been handling you people as tender as babies, because I had to because you're such important people, but now it's different. On killing Boone all of you might have been innocent, but now I know one of you isn't. One of you killed that woman, and it's a fair guess that the same one killed Boone. I—"

"Excuse me, Inspector." Frank Thomas Erskine was sharp, by no means apologetic, but neither was he outraged. "You've made a statement that you may regret. What about the man seen by Mr. Winterhoff running from the areaway—"

"Yeah, I've heard about him." Cramer was conceding nothing. "For the present I stick to my statement. I add to it that the Police Commissioner has just confirmed my belief that I'm in charge here, at the scene of a murder with those present detained, and the more time you waste bellyaching the longer you'll stay. Your families have been notified where you are and why. One of you thinks he can have me sent up for twenty years because I won't let him phone all his friends and lawyers. Okay. He don't phone."

Cramer made a face at them, at least it looked like it to me, and growled, "Do you understand the situation?"

Nobody answered. He went on, "Here's what I came in here to say. The piece of pipe she was killed with has been examined for fingerprints. We haven't found any that are any good. The galvanizing was rough to begin with, and it's a used piece of pipe, very old, and the galvanizing is flaking off, and there are blotches of stuff, paint and other matter, more or less all over it. We figure that anybody grasping that pipe hard enough to crack a skull with it would almost certainly get particles of stuff in the creases of his hands. I don't mean flakes you could see, I mean particles too small to be visible, and you wouldn't get them all out of the creases just by rubbing your palms on your clothes. The examination would have to be made with a microscope. I don't want to take all of you down to the laboratory, so I'm having a microscope brought here. I am requesting all of you to permit this examination of your hands, and also of your gloves and handkerchiefs."

Mrs. Boone spoke up, "But, Inspector, I've washed my hands. I went to the kitchen to help make sandwiches, and of course I washed my hands."

"That's too bad," Cramer growled. "We can still try it. Some of those particles might not come out of the creases even with washing. You can give your answers, yes or no, to Sergeant Stebbins. I'm busy."

He marched out and returned to the dining room. It was at that point that I felt I needed some arranging inside, and went to the office and told Wolfe I would be in my room if he wanted me. I stayed there over half an hour. It was one A.M. when the microscope came. Police cars were coming and going all the time, and it was by accident that, through my window, I saw a man get out of one carrying a large box. I gulped the rest of the milk and returned downstairs.

21.

I MIGHT as well have stayed put, because that was where the hand inspecting was done, my bedroom. The laboratory man wanted a quiet spot, and there was still activity everywhere else except Wolfe's room, which, by his instructions, was not to be entered. So the customers, one by one, had to climb the two flights. The apparatus, with its special light plugged in, was set up on my table. There were five of us in the room: the two experts, the dick who brought and took the customers, the current customer, and me sitting on the edge of the bed.

I was there partly because it was my room and I didn't care for the idea of abandoning it to a gang of strangers, and partly because I was stubborn and still couldn't understand why I was unable to pick the face, as I had greeted them at the door, of the one who had just finished killing Phoebe. That was the reason I might have bid as high as a nickel for Winterhoff's man in dark clothes darting and dashing. I wanted another good look at them. I had a feeling, of which I wouldn't have told Wolfe, that if I looked straight at the face of the person who had killed Phoebe, I would know it. It was an entirely new slant on crime detection, especially for me, but I had it. So I sat on the edge of my bed and looked straight at faces while the experts looked at hands.

First, Nina Boone. Pale, tired, and nervous.

Second, Don O'Neill. Resentful, impatient, and curious. Eyes bloodshot.

Third, Hattie Harding. Saggy and very jittery. Eyes nothing like as competent as they had been four days earlier in her office.

Fourth, Winterhoff. Distinguished, sweaty, and worried stiff.

Fifth, Father Erskine. Tense and determined.

Sixth, Alger Kates. Grim and about ready to cry. Eyes backing into his head.

Seventh, Mrs. Boone. Everything coming loose but trying to hang on. The tiredest of all.

Eighth, Solomon Dexter. Sort of swollen, with bags under the eyes. Not worried, but extremely resolute.

Ninth, Breslow. Lips tight with fury and eyes like a mad pig. He was the only one who stared back at me instead of at his own hand, under the light and the lens.

Tenth, Ed Erskine. Sarcastic, skeptical, and hangover all gone. About as worried as a pigeon in the park.

There had been no exclamations of delighted discovery from the experts, any more than from me. They had spoken to the customers, to instruct them about holding still and shifting position when required, and had exchanged brief comments in undertones, and that was all. They had tweezers and pill-boxes and other paraphernalia handy, but had made no use of it. When the last one, Ed Erskine, had been escorted out, I asked them:

"Any soap?"

The one without much chin replied, "We report to the Inspector."

"Goodness gracious," I said enviously. "It must be wonderful to be connected with the Police Department, with all the secrets. Why do you think Cramer let me come up and sit here and watch? To keep my mind a blank?"

"No doubt," the other one, the one with a jaw, said primly, "the Inspector will inform you of our findings. Go down and report, Phillips."

I was beginning to get restless, so, deciding to leave my room to its fate temporarily, I followed Phillips downstairs. If it was a weird experience for me, all these aliens trampling all over the house as if they owned it, I could imagine what the effect must be on Wolfe. Phillips trotted into the dining room, but Cramer wasn't among those present, and I steered him into the office. Wolfe was at his desk, and the P.C., the D.A., and the two FBI's were still there, all with their eyes on Cramer, who stood talking to them. He stopped at sight of Phillips

"Well?"

"On the microscopic examination of hands the results are negative, Inspector."

"The hell they are. Another big rousing achievement. Tell Stebbins to get all gloves and handkerchiefs from their persons and send them up to you. Including the ladies' bags.

Tell him to tag everything. Also from their overcoat pockets —no, send up coats and hats and all, and you see what's in the pockets. For God's sake don't mix anything up."

"Yes, sir." Phillips turned and went.

Not seeing how any good could come of staring straight at the faces of gloves and handkerchiefs, I crossed over to the Police Commissioner and addressed him:

"If you don't mind, this is my chair."

He looked startled, opened his mouth, shut it again, and moved to another seat. I sat down where I belonged. Cramer talked:

"You can do it if you can get away with it, but you know what the law is. Our jurisdiction extends to the limits of the premises occupied by the deceased provided it was the scene of the crime, but not otherwise. We can—"

"That's not the law," the D.A. snapped.

"You mean it's not statute But it's accepted custom and it's what thc courts stand for, so it's law for me. You wanted my opinion, and that's it. I won't be responsible for continued occupation of the apartment Miss Gunther was staying in, and not by my men anyway because I can't spare them. The tenant of the apartment is Kates. Three good searchers have spent an hour and a half there and haven't found anything. I'm willing to let them keep at it all night, or at least until we turn Kates loose, if and when we're through here, but any order for continued occupancy and keeping Kates out"— he looked at the P.C.—"will have to come from you, sir, or," he looked at the D.A., "from you."

Travis of the FBI put in, "I'd advise against it."

"This," the D.A. said stiffly, "is a local problem."

They went on. I started kicking my left ankle with my right foot, and vice versa. Wolfe was leaning back in his chair with his eyes closed, and I was pleased to note that his opinion of high strategy was apparently the same as mine. The P.C., the D.A., and the FBI, not to mention the head of the Homicide Squad, debating where Alger Kates was going to sleep, when he got a chance to sleep, and that after three cops had had the apartment all to themselves long enough to saw all the legs off the chairs and glue them back on. It developed that it was the D.A. who was plugging for continued occupancy. I decided to enter the conversation just for the hell of it and was considering which side to be on when the phone rang.

It was from Washington, for FBI Travis, and he came to my desk to take it. The others stopped talking and looked at him. On his part it was mostly listening. When he had finished he shoved the phone back and turned to announce:

"This has some bearing on what we've been discussing. Our

men and the Washington police have completed their search of Miss Gunther's apartment in Washington—one large room, bath, and kitchenette. In a hatbox on a shelf in a closet they found nine Stenophone cylinders—"

"Confound it!" Wolfe burst out. "Nine?" He was as indignant and irritated as if he had been served a veal cutlet with an egg perched on it. Everyone stared at him.

"Nine," said Travis curtly. He was justifiably annoyed at having his scene stolen. "Nine Stenophone cylinders. A BPR man was with them, and they are now at the BPR office running them off and making a transcription." He looked coldly at Wolfe. "What's wrong with nine?"

"For you," Wolfe said offensively, "apparently nothing. For me, nine is no better than none. I want ten."

"That's a damn shame. I apologize. They should have found ten." Having demolished Wolfe, he reported to the others, "They'll call again as soon as they get something we might use."

"Then they won't call," Wolfe declared, and shut his eyes again, leaving the discussion of the new development to the others. He was certainly being objectionable, and it wasn't hard to guess why. The howling insolence of committing a murder on his own stoop would alone have been enough, but in addition to that his house was filled from top to bottom with uninvited guests and he was absolutely powerless. That was dead against his policy, his practice, and his personality. Seeing that he was really in a bad way, and thinking it might be a good plan for him to keep himself at least partially informed of what was going on, since he was supposed to have an interest in the outcome, I went to the kitchen to get some beer for him. Evidently he was in too bad a humor even to remember to send for beer, since there were no signs of any.

Fritz and about a dozen assorted dicks were there drinking coffee. I told them:

"You sure are cluttering up the place, but I don't blame you. It isn't often that members of the lower clahsses get a chance to drink coffee made by Fritz Brenner."

There was a subdued, but close to unanimous, concert of Bronx cheers. One said, "Goodwin the gentleman. One, two, three, laugh."

Another said, "Hey, you know everything. What's the low-down on this NIA-BPR stuff? Is it a feud or not?"

I was putting six bottles and six glasses on a tray, with Fritz's help. "I'm glad to explain," I said generously. "The NIA and the BPR are in one respect exactly like the glorious PD, or Police Department. They have esprit de corps. Repeat it after me—no, don't bother. That is a French term, the language spoken by Frenchmen, the people who live in France, the literal translation of which is 'spirit of the body.' In our language we have no precise equivalent—"

The cheers had begun again, and the tray was ready, so I left them. Fritz came to the hall with me, closed the kitchen door, held my sleeve, and told my ear:

"Archie, this is awful. I just want to say I know how awful it is for you. Mr. Wolfe told me when I took up his breakfast this morning that you had formed a passion for Miss Gunther and she had you wound around her finger. She was a beautiful girl, very beautiful. This is awful, what happened here."

I said, "Go to hell," jerked my arm to free my sleeve, and took a step. Then I turned to him and said, "All I meant was, this is a hell of a night and it will take you a week to clean up the joint. Go back and finish that lesson in French I was giving them."

In the office they were as before. I peddled beer around, making three sales to outsiders, leaving three bottles for Wolfe, which was about as I had calculated, went back to the kitchen and got myself a sandwich and a glass of milk, and returned to my desk with them. The strategy council was going on and on, with Wolfe still aloof in spite of the beer. The sandwich made me hungry and I went and got two more. Long after they were gone the council was still chewing the fat.

They were handicapped, of course, by continual interruptions, both by phone and by personal appearances. One of the phone calls was for Travis from Washington, and when he was through with it his face displayed no triumph. The nine cylinders had all been listened to, and there was nothing for us to bite on. They contained plenty of evidence that they had been dictated by Boone at his Washington office on Tuesday afternoon, but no evidence at all that would help to uncover a murderer. The BPR was trying to hang onto the transcriptions, but the Washington FBI promised to send a copy to Travis, and he agreed to let Cramer see it.

"So," Travis said aggressively, daring us to hint that we were no better off than before, "that proves that Miss Gunther was lying about them She had them all the time."

"Nine." Wolfe grunted in disgust. "Pfui."

That was his only contribution to their discussion of the cylinders.

It was five minutes past three Tuesday morning when Phillips, the expert with less than his share of chin, entered the office with objects in his hands. In his right was a gray topcoat, and in his left was a silk scarf with stripes of dark brown and terra cotta. It was obvious that even an expert is capable of having feelings. His face showed plainly that he had something.

He looked at Wolfe and me and asked, "Do I report here, Inspector?"

"Go ahead." Cramer was impatient. "What is it?"

"This scarf was in the right-hand pocket of this coat. It was folded as it is now. Unfolding one fold exposes about forty square inches of its surface. On that surface are between fifteen and twenty particles of matter which in our opinion came from that piece of pipe. That is our opinion. Laboratory tests—"

"Sure." Cramer's eyes were gleaming. "You can test from hell to breakfast. You've got a microscope up there, and you know what I want right now. Is it good enough to act on, or isn't it?"

"Yes, sir it is. We made sure before—"

"Whose coat is it?"

"The tag say Alger Kates."

"Yeah," I agreed. "That's Kates's coat."

22.

SINCE they were a strategy council, naturally they didn't send for Kates immediately. They had to decide on strategy first—whether to circle him and get him tangled, or slide it into him gently, or just hit him on the head with it. What they really had to decide was who was going to handle it; that would determine the method, and they started to wrangle about it. The point was, as it always is when you've got a crusher like that scarf in his pocket, which way of using it was most likely to crumble him and get a confession? They hadn't been going long when Travis interposed:

"With all this top authority present, and me not in it officially anyhow, I hesitate to make a suggestion."

"So what is it?" the D.A. asked tartly.

"I would suggest Mr. Wolfe for it. I have seen him operate, and if it means anything I freely admit that he is my superior at it."

"Suits me," Cramer said at once.

The other two looked at each other. Neither liked what he

was looking at, and neither liked Travis's suggestion, so simultaneously they said nothing.

"Okay," Cramer said, "let's go. Where do you want the coat and scarf, Wolfe, in sight?"

Wolfe half opened his eyes. "What is this gentleman's name?"

"Oh. Phillips. Mr. Wolfe, Mr. Phillips."

"How do you do, sir. Give the coat to Mr Goodwin. Archie, put it behind the cushions on the couch. Give me the scarf, please."

Phillips had handed me the coat without hesitation, but now he balked. He looked at Cramer. "This is vital evidence. If those particles get brushed off and scattered . . ."

"I'm not a ninny," Wolfe snapped.

"Let him have it," Cramer said.

Phillips hated to do it. He might have been a mother instructed to entrust her newborn infant to a shady character. But he handed it over.

"Thank you, sir. All right, Mr. Cramer, get him in here."

Cramer went, taking Phillips with him. In a moment he was back, without Phillips and with Alger Kates. We all gazed at Kates as he stepped across and took the chair indicated by Cramer, facing Wolfe, but it didn't visibly disconcert him. He looked to me as he had up in my room, as if he might bust out crying any minute, but there was no evidence that he had done so. After he had sat down all I had was his profile.

"You and I have hardly spoken, have we, Mr. Kates?" Wolfe asked.

Kates's tongue came out to wet his lips and went back in again. "Enough to satisfy—" he began, but his thin voice threatened to become only a squeak, and he stopped for a second and then started over. "Enough to satisfy me."

"But my dear sir." Wolfe was gently reproachful. "I don't believe we've exchanged a word."

Kates did not unbend. "Haven't we?" he asked.

"No, sir. The devil of it is that I can't honestly say that I don't sympathize with your attitude. If I were in your position, innocently or not, I would feel the same. I don't like people piling questions on me, and in fact I don't tolerate it." Wolfe let his eyes open another millimeter. "By the way, I am now, momentarily, official. These gentlemen in authority have deputized me to talk with you. As you doubtless know, that doesn't mean that you *must* tolerate it. If you tried to leave this house before they let you go, you would be arrested as a material witness and taken somewhere, but you can't be compelled to take part in a conversation if you are determined not to. What do you say? Shall we talk?"

"I'm listening," Kates said.

"I know you are. Why?"

"Because, if I don't, the inference will be made that I'm frightened, and the further inference will be made that I am guilty of something that I am trying to conceal."

"Good. Then we understand each other." Wolfe sounded as if he were grateful for a major concession. With casual unhurried movement he brought the scarf out from beneath the rim of the desk, where he had been holding it in his hand, and put it down on the blotter. Then he cocked his head at Kates as if trying to decide where to begin. From where I sat, having Kates's profile, I couldn't tell whether he even gave the scarf a glance. Certainly he didn't turn pale or exhibit any hand-clenching or tremors of the limbs.

"On the two occasions," Wolfe said, "that Mr. Goodwin went to Fifty-fifth Street to see Miss Gunther, you were there. Were you a close friend of hers?"

"Not a close personal friend, no. In the past six months, since I've been doing confidential research directly under Mr. Boone, I've seen her frequently in connection with the work."

"Yet she was staying in your apartment."

Kates looked at Cramer. "You people have gone over this with me a dozen times."

Cramer nodded. "That's the way it goes, son. This'll make thirteen."

Kates returned to Wolfe. "The present housing shortage makes it extremely difficult, and often impossible, to get a room in a hotel. Miss Gunther could have used her position and connections to get a room, but that is against BPR policy, and also she didn't do things like that. A bed in a friend's apartment was available to me, and my wife was away. I offered the use of my apartment to Miss Gunther coming up on the plane from Washington, and she accepted."

"Had she ever stayed there before?"

"No."

"You had see her frequently for six months. What did you think of her?"

"I thought well of her."

"Did you admire her?"

"Yes. As a colleague."

"Did she dress well?"

"I never noticed particularly—no, that isn't true." Kates's voice zoomed for a squeak again and he used the controls. "If you think these questions are important and you want full and truthful answers. Considering Miss Gunther's striking appearance and her voluptuous figure, I thought she dressed extremely well for one in her position."

If Phoebe was here, I thought, she'd tell him he talks like an old-fashioned novel.

"Then," Wolfe said, "you did notice what she wore. In that case, when did you last see her wearing this scarf?" He used a thumb to indicate it.

Kates leaned forward to look at it. "I don't remember ever seeing her wear that. I never did." He settled back.

"That's strange." Wolfe was frowning. "This is important, Mr. Kates. Are you sure?"

Kates leaned forward again, saying, "Let me see it," and reached a hand for it.

Wolfe's hand was there before his, closing on it. "No," Wolfe said, "this will be an exhibit in a murder trial and therefore should not be handled indiscriminately." He stretched an arm to give Kates a closer look. Kates peered at it a moment, then leaned back and shook his head.

"I've never seen it before," he declared. "On Miss Gunther or anybody else."

"That's a disappointment," Wolfe said regretfully. "However, it doesn't exhaust the possibilities. You might have seen it before and now not recognize it because your previous view of it was in a dim light, for instance on the stoop of this house at night. I suggest that for your consideration, because clinging to this scarf are many tiny particles which came from the piece of pipe, showing that the scarf was used as a protection in clutching the pipe, and also because the scarf was found in the pocket of your overcoat."

Kates blinked at him. "Whose overcoat?"

"Yours. Get it, Archie." I went for it, and stood beside Kates, holding it by the collar, hanging full length. Wolfe asked, "That's your coat, isn't it?"

Kates sat and stared at the coat. Then he arose, turned his back on Wolfe, and called at the top of his voice, "Mr. Dexter! *Mr. Dexter! Come in here!*"

"Cut it out." Cramer was up and had him by the arm on the other side. "Cut out the yelling! What do you want Dexter for?"

"Then get him in here. If you want me to stop yelling, get him in here." Kates's voice was trembling. "I told him something like this would happen! I told Phoebe to have nothing to do with Nero Wolfe! I told her not to come here tonight! I—"

Cramer pounced. "When did you tell her not to come here tonight? When?"

Kates didn't answer. He realized his arm was being gripped,

looked down at Cramer's hand gripping it, and said, "Let go of me. Let go!" Cramer did so. Kates walked across to a chair against the wall, sat on it, and clamped his jaw. He was breaking off relations.

I said to Cramer, "If you want it, I was there when Rowcliffe was questioning him. He said he was at his friend's apartment on Eleventh Street, where he's staying, and Miss Gunther phoned to say she had just been told to come here and wanted to know if he had been told too, and he said yes but he wasn't coming and he tried to persuade her not to come, and when she said she was going to he decided to come too. I know you're busy, but if you don't read reports you throw wild punches."

I turned to include them all. "And if you want my opinion, with no fee, that's not Miss Gunther's scarf because it's not her style. She wouldn't have worn that thing. And it doesn't belong to Kates. Look at him. Gray suit, gray topcoat. Also a gray hat. I've never seen him in anything but gray, and if he was still speaking to us you could ask him."

Cramer strode to the door which connected with the front room, opened it a crack, and commanded, "Stebbins! Come in here."

Purley came at once. Cramer told him, "Take Kates to the dining room. Bring the others in here one at a time, and as we finish with them take them to the dining room."

Purley went with Kates, who didn't seem reluctant to go. In a moment another dick entered with Mrs. Boone. She wasn't invited to sit down. Cramer met her in the middle of the room, displayed the scarf, told her to take a good look at it but not to touch it, and then asked if she had ever seen it before. She said she hadn't, and that was all. She was led out and Frank Thomas Erskine was led in, and the performance was repeated. There were four more negatives, and then it was Winterhoff's turn.

With Winterhoff, Cramer didn't have to finish his speech. He showed the scarf and started, "Mr. Winterhoff, please look—"

"Where did you get that?" Winterhoff demanded, reaching for it. "That's my scarf!"

"Oh." Cramer backed up a step with it. "That's what we've been trying to find out. Did you wear it here tonight, or have it in your pocket?"

"Neither one. I didn't have it. That's the one that was stolen from me last week."

"Where and when last week?"

"Right here. When I was here Friday evening."

"Here at Wolfe's house?"

"Yes."

"You wore it here?"

"Yes."

"When you found it was gone, who helped you look for it? Who did you complain to?"

"I didn't—what's this all about? Who had it? Where did you get it?"

"I'll explain in a minute. I'm asking now, who did you complain to?"

"I didn't complain to anybody. I didn't notice it was gone until I got home. If—"

"You mentioned it to no one at all?"

"I didn't mention it here. I didn't know it was gone. I must have mentioned it to my wife—of course I did, I remember. But I have—"

"Did you phone here the next day to ask about it?"

"No, I didn't!" Winterhoff had been forcing himself to submit to the pressure. Now he was through. "Why would I? I've got two dozen scarves! And I insist that—"

"Okay, insist." Cramer was calm but bitter. "Since it's your scarf and you've been questioned about it, it is proper to tell you that there is evidence, good evidence, that it was wrapped around the pipe that Miss Gunther was killed with. Have you any comment?"

Winterhoff's face was moist with sweat, but it had already been that way up in my room when they were examining his hands. It was interesting that the sweat didn't seem to make him look any less distinguished, but it did detract some when he goggled, as he now did at Cramer. It occurred to me that his best friend ought to warn him not to goggle.

He finally spoke. "What's the evidence?"

"Particles from the pipe found on the scarf. Many of them, at one spot."

"Where did you find it?"

"In an overcoat pocket."

"Whose coat?"

Cramer shook his head. "You're not entitled to that. I'd like to ask you not to do any broadcasting on this, but of course you will." He turned to the dick. "Take him to the dining room and tell Stebbins not to bring any more in."

Winterhoff had things to say, but he was shooed out. When the door was closed behind him and the dick, Cramer sat down and put his palms on his knees, pulled in a deep breath, and expelled it noisily.

"Jee-zuss—Christ," he remarked.

23.

THERE was a long silence. I looked at the wall clock. It said two minutes to four. I looked at my wrist watch. It said one minute to four. In spite of the discrepancy it seemed safe to conclude that it would soon be four o'clock. From beyond the closed doors to the front room and the hall came faint suggestions of little noises, just enough to keep reminding us that silence wouldn't do. Every little noise seemed to be saying, come on, it's getting late, work it out. The atmosphere there in the office struck me as both discouraged and discouraging. Some buoyancy and backbone were needed.

"Well," I said brightly, "we've taken a big step forward. We have eliminated Winterhoff's darting and dashing man. I am prepared to go on the stand and swear that he didn't dash into the hall."

That got a rise out of nobody, which showed the pathetic condition they were in. All that happened was that the D.A. looked at me as if I reminded him of someone who hadn't voted for him.

The P.C. spoke. "Winterhoff is a damned liar. He didn't see a man running away from that stoop. He made that up."

"For God's sake," the D.A. burst out ferociously, "we're not after a liar! We're after a murderer!"

"I would like," Wolfe muttered sulkily, "to go to bed. It's four o'clock and you're stuck."

"Oh, we are." Cramer glowered at him. *"We're* stuck. The way you put it. I suppose *you're* not stuck?"

"Me? No, Mr. Cramer. No indeed. But I'm tired and sleepy."

That might have led to violence if there hadn't been an interruption. There was a knock on the door and a dick entered, approached Cramer, and reported:

"We've got two more taxi drivers, the two that brought Mrs. Boone and O'Neill. I thought you might want to see them, Inspector. One is named—"

He stopped on account of Cramer's aspect. "This," Cramer said, "will make you a Deputy Chief Inspector. Easy." He pointed to the door. "Out that way and find someone to tell it to." The dick, looking frustrated, turned and went. Cramer said to anyone who cared to listen, "My God. Taxi drivers!"

The P.C. said, "We'll have to let them go."

"Yes, sir," Cramer agreed. "I know we will. Get 'em in here, Archie."

So that was the state of mind the Inspector was in. As I proceeded to obey his command I tried to remember another occasion on which he had called me Archie, and couldn't, in all the years I had known him. Of course after he had got some sleep and had a shower he would feel differently about it, but I put it away for some fitting moment in the future to remind him that he had called me Archie. Meanwhile Purley and I, with plenty of assistance, herded everybody from the front room and dining room into the office.

The strategy council had left their chairs and collected at the far end of Wolfe's desk, standing. The guests took seats. The city employees, over a dozen of them, scattered around the room and stood looking as alert and intelligent as the facts of the case would permit, under the eye of the big boss, the P.C. himself.

Cramer, on his feet confronting them, spoke:

"We're letting you people go home. But before you go, this is the situation. The microscopic examination of your hands didn't show anything. But the microscope got results. On a scarf that was in a pocket of one of your overcoats, hanging in the hall, particles from the pipe were found. The scarf was unquestionably used by the murderer to keep his hand from contact with the pipe. Therefore—"

"Whose coat was it in?" Breslow blurted.

Cramer shook his head. "I'm not going to tell you whose coat it was or who the scarf belongs to, and I think it would be better if the owners didn't tell, because it would be sure to get to the papers, and you know what the papers—"

"No, you don't," Alger Kates piped up. "That would suit your plans, you and Nero Wolfe and the NIA, but you're not going to put any gag on me! It was my coat! And I've never seen the scarf before! This is the most—"

"That's enough, Kates," Solomon Dexter rumbled at him.

"Okay." Cramer did not sound displeased. "So it was found in Mr. Kates's coat, and he says he never saw the scarf before. That—"

"The scarf," Winterhoff interposed, his voice heavier and flatter than ever, "belongs to me. It was stolen from my overcoat in this house last Friday night. I haven't seen it since, until you showed it to me here. Since you have permitted Kates to make insinuations about the plans of the NIA—"

"No," Cramer said curtly, "that's out. I'm not interested in insinuations. If you people want to carry on your quarrel you can hire a hall. What I want to say is this, that some hours ago I said that one of you killed Miss Gunther, and

Mr. Erskine objected. Now there's no room for objection. Now there's no doubt about it. We could take you all down and book you as material witnesses. But being who you are, within a few hours you'd all be out on bail. So we're letting you go home, including the one who committed a murder here tonight, because we don't know which one it is. We intend to find out. Meanwhile you may be expected to be called on or sent for any time, day or night. You are not to leave the city, even for an hour, without permission. Your movements may or may not be kept under observation. That's up to us, and no protests about it will get you anywhere."

Cramer scanned the faces. "Police cars will take you home. You can go now, but one last word. This isn't going to let up. It's bad for all of you, and it will go on being bad until the murderer is caught. So if any of you knows anything that will help, the worst mistake you can make is not to let us have it. Stay now and tell us. The Police Commissioner and the District Attorney and I are right here and you can talk with any of us."

His invitation wasn't accepted, at least not on the terms as stated. The Erskine family lingered to exchange words with the D.A., Winterhoff had a point to make with the P.C., Mrs. Boone got Travis of the FBI, whom she apparently knew, to one side, Breslow had something to say to Wolfe, and Dexter confronted Cramer with questions. But before long they had all departed, and it didn't appear that anything useful had been contributed to the cause.

Wolfe braced his palms against the rim of his desk, pushed his chair back, and got to his feet.

Cramer, on the contrary, sat down. "Go to bed if you want to," he said grimly, "but I'm having a talk with Goodwin." Already it was Goodwin again. "I want to know who besides Kates had a chance to put that scarf in his coat."

"Nonsense." Wolfe was peevish. "With an ordinary person that might be necessary, but Mr. Goodwin is trained, competent, reliable, and moderately intelligent. If he could help on that he would have told us so. Merely ask him a question. I'll ask him myself. —Archie. Is your suspicion directed at anyone putting the scarf in the coat, or can you eliminate anyone as totally without opportunity?"

"No sir twice," I told him. "I've thought about it and gone over all of them. I was moving in and out between bell rings, and so were most of them. The trouble is the door to the front room was standing open, and so was the door from the front room to the hall."

Cramer grunted. "I'd give two bits to know how you would

have answered that question if you had been alone with Wolfe, and how you will answer it."

"If that's how you feel about it," I said, "you might as well skip it. My resistance to torture is strongest at dawn, which it is now, and how are you going to drag the truth out of me?"

"I could use a nap," G. G. Spero said, and he got the votes.

But what with packing the scarf in a box as if it had been a museum piece, which incidentally it now is, and collecting papers and miscellaneous items, it was practically five o'clock before they were finally out.

The house was ours again. Wolfe started for the elevator. I still had to make the rounds to see what was missing and to make sure there were no public servants sleeping under the furniture. I called to Wolfe:

"Instructions for the morning, sir?"

"Yes!" he called back. "Let me alone!"

24.

FROM there on I had a feeling that I was out of it. As it turned out, the feeling was not entirely justified, but anyhow I had it.

What Wolfe tells me, and what he doesn't tell me, never depends, as far as I can make out, on the relevant circumstances. It depends on what he had to eat at the last meal, what he is going to have to eat at the next meal, the kind of shirt and tie I am wearing, how well my shoes are shined, and so forth. He does not like purple. Once Lily Rowan gave me a dozen Sulka shirts, with stripes of assorted colors and shades. I happened to put on the purple one the day we started on the Chesterton-Best case, the guy that burgled his own house and shot a week-end guest in the belly. Wolfe took one look at the shirt and clammed up on me. Just for spite I wore the shirt a week, and I never did know what was going on, or who was which, until Wolfe had it all wrapped up, and even then I had to get most of the details from the newspapers and Dora Chesterton, with whom I had struck up an acquaintance. Dora had a way of—no, I'll save that for my autobiography.

The feeling that I was out of it had foundation in fact. Tuesday morning Wolfe breakfasted at the usual hour—my deduction from this evidence, that Fritz took up his tray, loaded, at eight o'clock, and brought it down empty at ten minutes to nine. On it was a note instructing me to tell Saul Panzer and Bill Gore, when they phoned in, to report at the office at eleven o'clock, and furthermore to arrange for Del Bascom, head of the Bascom Detective Agency, also to be present. They were all there waiting for him when he came down from the plant rooms, and he chased me out. I was sent to the roof to help Theodore cross-pollinate. When I went back down at lunch time Wolfe told me that envelopes from Bascom were to reach him unopened.

"Hah," I said. "Reports? Big operations?"

"Yes." He grimaced. "Twenty men. One of them may be worth his salt."

There went another five hundred bucks a day up the flue. At that rate the NIA retainer wouldn't last long.

"Do you want me to move to a hotel?" I inquired. "So I won't hear anything unfit for my ears?"

He didn't bother to answer. He never let himself get upset just before a meal if he could help it.

I could not, of course, be really blackballed, no matter what whim had struck him. For one thing, I had been among those present, and was therefore in demand. Friends on papers, especially Lon Cohen of the *Gazette,* thought I ought to tell them exactly who would be arrested and when and where. And Tuesday afternoon Inspector Cramer decided there was work to be done on me and invited me to Twentieth Street. He and three others did the honors. What was eating him was logic. To this effect: The NIA was Wolfe's client. Therefore, if I had seen any NIA person lingering unnecessarily in the neighborhood of Kates's overcoat as it hung in the hall, I would have reported it to Wolfe but not to anyone else. So far so good. Perfectly sound. But then Cramer went on to assume that with two hours of questions, back-tracking, leap-frogging, and ambushing, he and his bunch could squeeze it out of me, which was droll. Add to that, that there was nothing in me to squeeze, and it became quaint. Anyhow, they tried hard.

It appeared that Wolfe too thought I might still have uses. When he came down to the office at six o'clock he got into his chair, rang for beer, sat for a quarter of an hour, and then said:

"Archie."

It caught me in the middle of a yawn. After that was attended to I said:

"Yeah."

He was frowning at me. "You've been with me a long time now."

"Yeah. How shall we do it? Shall I resign, or shall you fire me, or shall we just call it off by mutual consent?"

He skipped that. "I have noted, perhaps in more detail than you think, your talents and capacities. You are an excellent observer, not in any respect an utter fool, completely intrepid, and too conceited to be seduced into perfidy."

"Good for me. I could use a raise. The cost of living has incr—"

"You eat and sleep here, and because you are young and vain you spend too much for your clothes." He gestured with a finger. "We can discuss that some other time. What I have in mind is a quality in you which I don't at all understand but which I know you have. Its frequent result is a willingness on the part of young women to spend time in your company."

"It's the perfume I use. From Brooks Brothers. They call it Stag at Eve." I regarded him suspiciously. "You're leading up to something. You've done the leading up. What's the something?"

"Find out how willing you can make Miss Boone, as quickly as possible."

I stared. "You know," I said reproachfully, "I didn't know that kind of a thought ever got within a million miles of you. Make Miss Boone? If you can think it you can do it. Make her yourself."

"I am speaking," he said coldly, "of an investigating operation by gaining her confidence."

"That way it sounds even worse." I continued to stare. "However, let's put the best possible construction on it. Do you want me to worm a confession out of her that she murdered her uncle and Miss Gunther? No, thanks."

"Nonsense. You know perfectly well what I want."

"Tell me anyway. What do you want?"

"I want information on these points. The extent of her personal or social contacts, if any, with anyone connected with the NIA, especially those who were here last night. The same for Mrs. Boone, her aunt. Also, how intimate was she with Miss Gunther, what did they think of each other, and how much did she see of Miss Gunther the past week? That would do to start. If developments warrant it, you can then get more specific. Why don't you telephone her now?"

"It seems legitimate," I conceded, "up to the point where we get specific, and that can wait. But do you mean to say you think one of those NIA specimens is it?"

"Why not? Why shouldn't he be?"

"It's so damn obvious."

"Bah. Nothing is obvious in itself. Obviousness is subjective. Three pursuers learn that a fugitive boarded a train for Philadelphia. To the first pursuer it's obvious that the fugitive has gone to Philadelphia. To the second pursuer it's obvious that he left the train at Newark and has gone somewhere else. To the third pursuer, who knows how clever the fugitive is, it's obvious that he didn't leave the train at Newark, because that would be too obvious, but stayed on it and went to Philadelphia. Subtlety chases the obvious up a never-ending spiral and never quite catches it. Do you know Miss Boone's telephone number?"

I might have suspected him of sending me outdoors to play, to keep me out of mischief, but for the fact that it was a nuisance for him to have me out of the house, since he either had to answer the phone himself or let Fritz interrupt his other duties to attend to both the phone and the doorbell. So I granted his good faith, at least tentatively, and swiveled my chair to dial the Waldorf's number, and asked for Mrs. Boone's room. The room answered with a male voice that I didn't recognize, and after giving my name, and waiting longer than seemed called for, I had Nina.

"This is Nina Boone. Is this Mr. Goodwin of Nero Wolfe's office? Did I get that right?"

"Yep. In the pay of the NIA. Thank you for coming to the phone."

"Why—you're welcome. Did you—want something?"

"Certainly I did, but forget it. I'm not calling about what I want or wanted, or could easily want. I'm calling about something somebody else wants, because I was asked to, only in my opinion he's cuckoo. You realize the position I'm in. I can't call you up and say this is Archie Goodwin and I just drew ten bucks from the savings bank and how about using it to buy dinner for two at that Brazilian restaurant on Fifty-second Street? What's the difference whether that's what I want to do or not, as long as I can't? Am I keeping you from something important?"

"No . . . I have a minute. What is it that somebody else wants?"

"I'll come to that. So all I can say is, this is Archie Goodwin snooping for the NIA, and I would like to use some NIA expense money to buy you a dinner at that Brazilian restaurant on Fifty-second Street, with the understanding that it is strictly business and I am not to be trusted. To give you an idea how tricky I am, some people look under the bed at night, but I look *in* the bed, to make sure I'm not already there laying for me. Is the minute up?"

"You sound really dangerous. Is that what somebody else wanted you to do, kid me into having dinner with you?"

"The dinner part was my idea. It popped out when I heard your voice again. As for somebody else—you appreciate that working on this thing I'm thrown in with all sorts of people, not only Nero Wolfe, who is—well, he can't help it, he's what he is—but also the police, the FBI, the District Attorney's outfit—all kinds. What would you say if I told you that one of them told me to call you and ask where Ed Erskine is?"

"Ed Erskine?" She was flabbergasted. "Ask *me* where Ed Erskine is?"

"That's right."

"I'd say he was out of his mind."

"So would I. So that's settled. Now before we hang up, to leave no loose ends hanging, maybe you'd better answer my own personally conducted question, about the dinner. How do you usually say no? Blunt? Or do you zigzag to avoid hurting people's feelings?"

"Oh, I'm blunt."

"All right, wait till I brace myself. Shoot."

"I couldn't go tonight, no matter how tricky you are. I'm eating here with my aunt in her room."

"Then supper later. Or breakfast. Lunch. Lunch tomorrow at one?"

There was a pause. "What kind of a place is this Brazilian restaurant?"

"Okay, out of the way, and good food."

"But . . . whenever I go on the street—"

"I know. That's how it is. Leave by the Forty-ninth Street entrance. I'll be there at the curb with a dark blue Wethersill sedan. I'll be right there from twelve-fifty on. You can trust me to be there, but beyond that, remember, be on your guard."

"I may be a little late."

"I should hope so. You look perfectly normal to me. And please don't, five or ten years from now, try to tell me that I said you look average. I didn't say average, I said normal. See you tomorrow."

As I pushed the phone back I had a notion that a gleam of self-congratulation might be visible in my eyes, so I didn't turn immediately to face Wolfe but found papers on my desk that needed attention. After a moment he muttered:

"This evening would have been better."

I counted ten. Then, still without turning, I said distinctly, "My dear sir, try getting her to meet *you* any time whatever, even at Tiffany's to try things on."

He chuckled. Before long he chuckled again. Finding that irritating, I went up to my room and kept busy until dinnertime straightening up. Fritz and Charley hadn't been able to get up that high on account of the condition of the rest of the house, and while the microscope experts had been neat and apparently respectable, I thought a spot inventory wouldn't do any harm.

Toward the end of dinner, with the salad and cheese, a little controversy arose. I wanted to have our coffee there in the dining room and then go straight up to bed, and Wolfe, while admitting that he too needed sleep, wanted the coffee in the office as usual. He got arbitrary about it, and just as an object lesson I sat tight. He went to the office and I stayed in the dining room. When I was through I went to the kitchen and told Fritz:

"I'm sorry you had that extra trouble, serving coffee in two places, but he has got to learn how to compromise. You heard me offer to split the difference and drink it in the hall."

"It was no trouble at all," Fritz said graciously. "I understand, Archie. I understand why you're being erratic. There goes the doorbell."

It was a temptation to let the damn thing ring. I needed sleep. So did Wolfe, and all I had to do was flip the switch there on the kitchen wall to stop the bell ringing. But I didn't flip it. I said to Fritz, "Justice. The public weal. Duty, goddam it," and went to the front and pulled the door open.

25.

THE guy standing there said, "Good evening. I would like to see Mr. Wolfe."

I had never seen him before. He was around fifty, medium-sized, with thin straight lips and the kind of eyes that play poker for blood. The first tenth of a second I thought he was one of Bascom's men, and then saw that his clothes ruled that out. They were quiet and conservative and must have had at least three try-ons. I told him:

"I'll see if he's in. Your name, please?"

"John Smith."

"Oh. What do you want to see him about, Mr. Jones?"

"Private and urgent business."

"Can you be more specific?"

"I can to him, yes."

"Good. Sit down and read a magazine."

I shut the door on him, clear shut, and went to the office and told Wolfe:

"Mr. John Smith, which he must have got out of a book, looks like a banker who would gladly lend you a dime on a cupful of diamonds. I left him on the stoop, but don't worry about him being insulted because he has no feelings. Please don't ask me to find out what he wants because it might take hours."

Wolfe grunted. "What is your opinion?"

"None at all. I am not being permitted to know where we're at. The natural impulse is to kick him off the stoop. I'll say this for him, he's not an errand boy."

"Bring him in."

I did so. In spite of his obnoxious qualities and of his keeping us up, I put him in the red leather chair because that had him facing both of us. He was not a lounger. He sat up straight, with his fingers intertwined in his lap, and told Wolfe:

"I gave the name of John Smith because my name is of no significance. I am merely an errand boy."

Starting off by contradicting me. He went on:

"This is a confidential matter and I must speak with you privately."

Wolfe shook his head. "Mr. Goodwin is my confidential assistant. His ears are mine. Go ahead."

"No." Smith's tone implied, and that settles it. "I have to be alone with you."

"Bah." Wolfe pointed to a picture of the Washington Monument, on the wall fifteen feet to his left. "Do you see that picture? It is actually a perforated panel. If Mr. Goodwin is sent from the room he will go to an alcove around a corner of the hall, across from the kitchen door, open the panel on that side, invisible to us, and watch us and listen to us. The objection to that is that he would be standing up. He might as well stay here sitting down."

Without batting an eye, Smith stood up. "Then you and I will go to the hall."

"No we won't.—Archie. Mr. Smith wants his hat and coat."

I arose and moved. When I was halfway across the room Smith sat down again. I whirled, returned to my base, and did likewise.

"Well, sir?" Wolfe demanded.

"We have somebody," Smith said, in what was apparently the only tone he ever used, "for the Boone and Gunther murders."

"We? Somebody?"

Smith untangled his fingers, raised a hand to scratch the side of his nose, dropped the hand, and retwined the fingers. "Of course," he said, "death is always a tragedy. It causes grief and suffering and often hardship. That cannot be avoided. But in this case, the deaths of these two people, it has already caused widespread injury to many thousands of innocent persons and created a situation that amounts to gross injustice. As you know, as we all know, there are elements in this country that seek to undermine the very foundations of our society. Death is serving them—*has* served them well. The very backbone of our free democratic system—composed of our most public-spirited citizens, our outstanding businessmen who keep things going for us—is in great and real peril. The source of that peril was an event—now two events—which may have resulted either from the merest chance or from deep and calculated malice. From the standpoint of the common welfare those two events were in themselves unimportant. But overwhelmingly—"

"Excuse me." Wolfe wiggled a finger at him. "I used to make speeches myself. The way I would put it, you're talking about the nation-wide reaction against the National Industrial Association on account of the murders. Is that correct?"

"Yes. I am emphasizing the contrast between the trivial character of the events in themselves and the enormous harm—"

"Please. You've made that point. Go on to the next one. But first tell me, do you represent the NIA?"

"No. I represent, actually, the founding fathers of this country. I represent the best and most fundamental interests of the American people. I—"

"All right. Your next point?"

Smith untwined his fingers again. This time it was the chin that needed scratching. When that was finished he proceeded, "The existing situation is intolerable. It is playing directly into the hands of the most dangerous and subversive groups and doctrines. No price would be too high to pay for ending it, and ending it at the earliest possible moment. The man who performed that service would deserve well of his country. He would earn the gratitude of his fellow citizens, and naturally, especially of those who are being made to suffer under this unjust odium."

"In other words," Wolfe suggested, "he ought to be paid something."

"He *would* be paid something."

"Then it's too bad I'm already engaged. I like being paid."

"There would be no conflict. The objectives are identical."

Wolfe frowned. "You know, Mr. Smith," he said admiringly, "I like the way you started this. You said it all, except certain details, in your first short sentence. Who are you and where do you come from?"

"That," Smith declared, "is stupid. You're not stupid. You can learn who I am, of course, if you want to take the time and trouble. But there are seven respectable—*very* respectable—men and women with whom I am playing bridge this evening. After a dinner party. Which accounts for the whole evening, from seven o'clock on."

"That should cover it adequately. Eight against two."

"Yes, it really should," Smith agreed. He untangled his fingers once more, but not to scratch. He reached to his side coat pocket and pulled out a package wrapped neatly in white paper and fastened with Scotch tape. It was big enough to be tight in his pocket and he had to use both hands. "As you say," he remarked, "there are certain details. The amount involved is three hundred thousand dollars. I have one-third of it here."

I gave it a look and decided it couldn't all be in hundreds. There must have been some five-hundreds and grands.

One of Wolfe's brows went up. "Since you're playing bridge this evening, and since you came here on the assumption that I'm a blackguard, isn't that a little foolhardy? Mr. Goodwin, as I told you, is my confidential assistant. What if he took that away from you and put it in the safe and saw you to the sidewalk?"

For the first time the expression of Smith's face changed, but the little crease that showed in his forehead didn't look like apprehension. "Perhaps," he said, and there was no change in his voice, "you're stupid after all, though I doubt it. We know your record and your character. There isn't the slightest assumption that you're a blackguard. You are being given an opportunity to perform a service—"

"No," Wolfe said positively. "We've had that."

"Very well. But that's the truth. If you ask why you're being paid so large a sum to perform it, here are the reasons. First, everybody knows that you get exorbitant fees for everything you do. Second, from the standpoint of the people who are paying you, the rapidly accumulating public disfavor, which is totally undeserved, is costing them or will cost them, directly or indirectly, hundreds of millions. Three hundred thousand dollars is a mere nothing. Third, you will have expenses, and they may be large. Fourth, we are aware of the difficulties involved, and I tell you frankly that we know of no one except you who can reasonably be expected to solve them. There is no assumption whatever that you're a blackguard. That remark was completely uncalled for."

"Then perhaps I misunderstood the sentence you started with." Wolfe's eyes were straight at him. "Didn't you say you have somebody for the Boone and Gunther murders?"

"Yes." Smith's eyes were straight back at him.

"Who have you?"

"The word 'have' was a little inexact. It might have been better to say we have somebody to suggest."

"Who?"

"Either Solomon Dexter or Alger Kates. We would prefer Dexter but Kates would do. We would be in a position to co-operate on certain aspects of the evidence. After your plans are made I'll confer with you on that. The other two hundred thousand, by the way, would not be contingent on conviction. You couldn't possibly guarantee that. Another third would be paid on indictment, and the last third on the opening day of the trial. The effect of indictment and trial would be sufficient, if not wholly satisfactory."

"Are you a lawyer, Mr. Smith?"

"Yes."

"Wouldn't you pay more for Dexter than for Kates? You should. He's the Acting Director of the Bureau of Price Regulation. It would be worth more to you."

"No. We made the amount large, even exorbitant, to exclude any bargaining." Smith tapped the package with his finger. "This is probably a record."

"Good heavens, no." Wolfe was mildly indignant, as if it had been intimated that his schooling had stopped at about the sixth grade. "There was Teapot Dome. I could rattle off eight, ten, a dozen instances. Alyattes of Lydia got the weight of ten panthers in gold. Richelieu paid D'Effiat a hundred thousand livres in one lump—the equivalent, at a minimum, of two million dollars today. No, Mr. Smith, don't flatter yourself that you're making a record. Considering what you're bidding for, you're a piker."

Smith was not impressed. "In cash," he said. "For you its equivalent, paid by check, would be around two million."

"That's right," Wolfe agreed, being reasonable. "Naturally that had occurred to me. I'm not pretending you're being niggardly." He sighed. "I'm no fonder of haggling than you are. But I may as well say it, there's an insuperable objection."

Smith blinked. I caught him at it. "What is it?"

"Your choice of targets. To begin with, they're too obvious, but the chief obstacle would be motive. It takes a good motive for a murder, and a really tiptop one for two murders. With either Mr. Dexter or Mr. Kates I'm afraid it simply couldn't be done, and I'll have to say definitely that I won't try it.

You have generously implied that I'm not a jackass, but I would be, if I undertook to get either Mr. Dexter or Mr. Kates indicted and tried, let alone convicted." Wolfe looked and sounded inflexible. "No, sir. But you might find someone who would at least attempt it. How about Mr. Bascom, of the Bascom Detective Agency? He's a good man."

"I have told you," Smith said, "that you'll get co-operation on evidence."

"No. The absence of adequate motive would make it impossible in spite of evidence, which would have to be circumstantial. Besides, considering the probable source of any evidence you would be able to produce, and since it would be directed against a BPR man, it would be suspect anyhow. You see that."

"Not necessarily."

"Oh, yes. Inevitably."

"No." Smith's face stayed exactly as before, though he had made a major decision, to show a card. He turned the card over without a flicker. "I'll give you an example. If the taxi driver who brought Dexter here testified that he saw him concealing a piece of iron pipe under his coat, with a scarf wrapped around it, that evidence wouldn't be suspect."

"Perhaps not," Wolfe conceded. "Have you got the taxi driver?"

"No. I was merely giving you an example. How could we go after the taxi driver, or anyone else, before we have come to an agreement on the—on a name?"

"You couldn't, of course. Have you any other examples?"

Smith shook his head. That was one way in which he resembled Wolfe. He didn't see any sense in using a hundred ergs when fifty would do the job. Wolfe's average on head-shaking was around an eighth of an inch to the right and the same distance to the left, and if you had attached a meter to Smith you would have got about the same result. However, Wolfe was still more economical on physical energy. He weighed twice as much as Smith, and therefore his expenditure per pound of matter, which is the only fair way to judge, was much lower.

"You're getting a little ahead," Smith stated. "I said we would confer on aspects of evidence after your plans are made. You will make plans only after you have accepted the offer. Do I understand that you've accepted it?"

"You do not. Not as described. I decline it."

Smith took it like a gentleman. He said nothing. After some long seconds of saying nothing, he swallowed, and that was his first sign of weakness. Evidently he was throwing in his hand and was ready for another deal. When, after another period of silence, he swallowed again, there was no question about it.

"There is another possibility," he said, "that would not be open to the objections you have made. Don O'Neill."

"M-m-m-m," Wolfe remarked.

"He also came in a taxicab. The motive is plain and in fact already established, since it is the motive that has already been accepted, wrongly and maliciously, all over the country. He would not serve the purpose as satisfactorily as Dexter or Kates, but it would transfer the public resentment from an institution or group to an individual; and that would change the picture completely."

"M-m-m-m."

"Also, evidence would not be suspect on account of its source."

"M-m-m-m."

"And therefore the scope of the evidence could be substantially widened. For example, it might be possible to introduce the testimony of a person or persons who saw, here in your hall, O'Neill putting the scarf into the pocket of Kates's overcoat. I understand that Goodwin, your confidential assistant, was there throughout—"

"No," Wolfe said curtly.

"He doesn't mean I wasn't there," I assured Smith with a friendly grin. "Only that I've already been too damn positive about it. You should have come sooner. I would have been glad to discuss terms. When O'Neill tried to buy me it was Sunday, and I can't be bribed on Sunday—"

His eyes darted at me and through me. "What did O'Neill want you to do?"

I shook my head. Probably a thousand ergs. "That wouldn't be fair. Would you want me to tell him what *you* wanted me to do?"

He was strongly tempted to insist, there was no doubt about his thirst for knowledge, but his belief in the conservation of energy, coupled with the opinion he had formed of me, won the day. He gave it up without another try and returned to Wolfe.

"Even if Goodwin couldn't give it," he said, "there is still a good chance of testimony to that effect being available."

"Not from Mr. Breslow," Wolfe declared. "He would be a wretched witness. Mr. Winterhoff would do fairly well. Mr. Erskine Senior would be admirable. Young Mr. Erskine—I don't know, I rather doubt it. Miss Harding would be the best of all. Could you get her?"

"You're going too fast again."

"Not at all. Fast? Such details are of the greatest importance."

"I know they are. *After* you are committed. Are you accepting my suggestion about O'Neill?"

"Well." Wolfe leaned back, opened his eyes to a wider slit, and brought his finger tips together at the apex of his central bulk. "I'll tell you, Mr. Smith. The best way to put it, I think, is in the form of a message, or rather messages, for Mr. Erskine. Tell Mr. Erskine—"

"I'm not representing Erskine. I have mentioned no names."

"No? I thought I heard you mention Mr. O'Neill, and Mr. Dexter and Mr. Kates. However, the difficulty is this, that the police or the FBI may find that tenth cylinder at any moment, and in all likelihood that would make fools of all of us."

"Not if we have—"

"Please, sir. You have talked. Let me talk. On the hypothesis that you may run across Mr. Erskine. Tell him that I am grateful for this suggestion regarding the size of the fee I may ask for without shocking him. I'll remember it when I make out my bill. Tell him that I appreciate his effort to pay the fee in a way that would keep it off my income tax report, but that form of skulduggery doesn't appeal to me. It's a matter of taste, and I happen not to like that. Tell him that I am fully aware that every minute counts; I know that the death of Miss Gunther has increased the public resentment to an unprecedented outburst of fury; I read the editorial in today's *Wall Street Journal;* I heard Raymond Swing on the radio this evening; I know what's happening."

Wolfe opened his eyes still wider. "Especially tell him this. If this idiotic flimflam is persisted in there will probably be the devil to pay and I'll be helpless, but I'll send in a bill just the same, and I'll collect it. I am now convinced that he is either a murderer or a simpleton, and possibly both. He is not, thank God, my client. As for you—no, I won't bother. As you say, you are merely an errand boy, and I suppose a reputable lawyer, of the highest standing. Therefore you are a sworn officer of the law Pfui!—Archie. Mr. Smith is going."

He had indeed left his chair and was upright. But he wasn't quite going. He said, in precisely the same tone he had used at the door when telling me he would like to see Mr. Wolfe:

"I would like to know whether I can count on this being treated as confidential. I merely want to know what to expect."

"You're a simpleton too," Wolfe snapped. "What's the difference whether I say yes or no—to you? I don't even know your name. Wouldn't I do as I please?"

"You think—" Smith said, and didn't finish it. Probably the sentence as conceived might have betrayed a trace of some emotion, like sizzling rage for instance, and that wasn't to be permitted under any circumstances. So I don't think it is exaggerating to say that he was rendered speechless. He stayed that way clear out to the stoop, not even telling me good night.

By the time I got back to the office Wolfe had already rung for beer. I knew that by deduction when Fritz entered almost immediately with the tray. I blocked him off and told him:

"Mr. Wolfe has changed his mind. Take it back. It's after ten o'clock, he had only two hours' sleep last night, and he's going to bed. So are you and either me or I or both."

Wolfe said nothing and made no sign, so Fritz beat it with the tray.

"It reminds me," I remarked, "of that old picture, there was one in our dining room out in Ohio, of the people in the sleigh throwing the baby out to the wolves that were chasing them. That may not strictly apply to Dexter or Kates, but it certainly does to O'Neill. Esprit de corps my eye. Good God, he was the Chairman of the Dinner Committee. I used to worry about that picture. One way of looking at it, it was heartless to toss out the baby, but on the other hand if they hadn't, the wolves would eventually have got the whole works, baby, horses, and all. Of course the man could have jumped out himself, or the woman could. I remember I decided that if it was me I would kiss the woman and baby good-by and then jump. I was eight years old at the time, a minor, and I don't regard myself as still committed to that. What do you think of the lousy bastards, anyhow?"

"They're in a panic." Wolfe stood up and pulled his vest down, and maneuvered himself into motion toward the door. "They're desperate. Good night, Archie." From the threshold he rumbled, without turning, "For that matter, so am I."

26.

THE next day, Wednesday, here came the envelopes from Bascom. There were four in the morning mail, three in the one o'clock delivery (as I was later informed for bookkeeping purposes, since I was not there at the time), and in late afternoon nine more arrived by messenger. At that time I hadn't the slightest idea what line the Bascom battalion was advancing on, nor did I know what Saul Panzer and Bill Gore were doing, since their telephoned reports were taken by Wolfe, with me instructed to disconnect. The Bascom envelopes were delivered to Wolfe unopened, as ordered.

I was being entrusted with nothing but the little chores, as for example a phone call I was told to make to the Stenophone Company to ask them to deliver a machine to us on a daily rental basis—one equipped with a loud-speaker, like the one the manager had brought us on Sunday and sent for on Monday. They weren't very affable about it and I had to be persuasive to get a promise of immediate delivery. I followed instructions and got the promise, though it was clear over my head, since we had nothing to play on it. An hour later the machine came and I stuck it in a corner.

The only other Wednesday morning activity in which I had a share was a phone call to Frank Thomas Erskine. I was told to make it, and did so, informing Erskine that expenses were skyrocketing and we wanted a check for another twenty thousand at his early convenience. He took that as a mere routine detail and came back at me for an appointment with Wolfe at eleven o'clock, which was made.

The most noteworthy thing about that was that when they—Breslow, Winterhoff, Hattie Harding, and the two Erskines—arrived, sharp at eleven, they had Don O'Neill with them! That was a fair indication that they had not come to take up where John Smith had left off, since Smith's central idea had been to frame O'Neill for a pair of murders, unless they were prepared to sweeten it up with an offer of a signed confession by O'Neill in triplicate, one copy for our files, and I felt that I knew O'Neill too well to expect anything like that, since he had tried to kick me.

Erskine brought the check with him. They stayed over an hour, and it was hard to guess why they had bothered to come, unless it was to show us in the flesh how harassed they were. No comment remotely touching on the errand of John Smith was made by anyone, including Wolfe. Half of their hour was used up in trying to get from Wolfe some kind of a progress report, which meant it was wasted, and they spent most of the other half in an attempt to pry a prognosis out of him. Twenty-four hours? Forty-eight? Three days? For God's sake, when? Erskine stated categorically that each additional day's delay meant untold damage to the most vital interests of the Republic and the American people.

"You're breaking my heart, Pop," young Erskine said sarcastically.

"Shut up!" his father barked at him.

They scratched and pulled hair right in front of us. The pressure was too much for them, and the NIA was no longer a united front. I sat and looked them over, having in mind

Smith's offer of testimony regarding the placing of the scarf in Kates's overcoat pocket, and came to the conclusion that it might be had from any one of them with respect to any other of them, with the possible exception of Erskine vs. Erskine, and even that was not unthinkable. Their only constructive contribution was the announcement that the next day, Thursday, over two hundred morning and evening papers in a hundred towns and cities would run a full page ad offering a reward of one hundred thousand dollars to anyone furnishing information leading to the arrest and trial of the murderer of either Cheney Boone or Phoebe Gunther, or both.

"There should be a healthy reaction to that, don't you think?" Erskine asked plaintively but not too hopefully.

I missed Wolfe's answer, and the rest of it, because I was leaving at that moment, on my way upstairs to run a comb through my hair and maybe wash my hands. I barely had time enough to get the car and be parked at the Forty-ninth Street entrance of the Waldorf at twelve-fifty, and since once in a million years a girl is early instead of late I didn't want to take a chance.

27.

NINA BOONE showed up at fourteen minutes past one, which was par and therefore called for no comment one way or the other. I met her as she emerged, steered her to where I was parked just west of the entrance, and opened the door. She climbed in. I turned to observe, and, as I expected, there one was, looking left and right. He was not an acquaintance and I didn't know his name, but I had seen him around. I crossed to him and said:

"I'm Archie Goodwin, Nero Wolfe's handy man. If you'd been on her heels you'd have seen her get in my car there. I can't ask you to ride with us because I'm working on her, but here's some choices. I'll wait till you get a taxi, and I'll bet you a finiff I lose you in less than ten minutes; or I'll grease you to miss the trail right here. Two bits. Fifteen cents now and the other dime when I see a copy of your report. If—"

"I've been told," he said, "that there are only two ways to deal with you. One is to shoot you, and this is too public. The other—give me the fifteen cents."

"Okay." I fished for three nickels and handed them to him.

"It's on the NIA. Actually I don't care. We're going to Ribeiro's, the Brazilian restaurant on Fifty-second Street."

I went and got in the car beside my victim, started the engine, and rolled.

A corner table in the side room at Ribeiro's is a good place to talk. The food is no great treat to one who gets fed by Fritz Brenner three times a day, but it goes down all right, there is no music, and you can wave a fork in any direction without stabbing anybody except your own companion.

"I don't believe," Nina said after we had ordered. "that anyone has recognized me. Anyhow no one is staring at me. I guess all obscure people think it would be wonderful to be a celebrity and have people look at you and point you out in restaurants and places. I know I did. Now I simply can't stand it. It makes me want to scream at them. Of course I might not feel that way if my picture had been in the papers because I was a movie star or because I had done something worth while—you know, remarkable."

So, I thought, she wanted someone besides Aunt Luella to talk to. Okay, let her talk.

"And yet," I told her, "you must have had your share of staring before this happened. You're not actually unsightly."

"No?" She didn't try to smile. "How do you know? The way I look now."

I inspected her. "It's a bad time to judge," I admitted. "Your eyes are puffy and you've been clamping your jaw so much that your chin juts. But still there's enough to go by for an estimate. The cheekbone curve is very nice, and the temples and forehead are way above the average. The hair, of course, has not been affected at all. Seeing you from behind on the sidewalk, one man out of three would walk faster to get a look at you from the side or the front."

"Oh? And the other two?"

"My lord," I protested, "what do you want for nothing? One out of three is tremendous. I was piling it on, merely because your hair happens to appeal to me and I might go so far as to break into a trot."

"Then next time I'll sit with my back to you." She moved her hand to her lap to make room for the waiter. "I've been wanting to ask you, and you've got to tell me, who was it that told you to ask me where Ed Erskine was?"

"Not yet. My rule with a girl is to spend the first fifteen minutes discussing her looks. There's always a chance I'll say something that appeals to her, and then it's smooth sailing. Besides, it wouldn't be in good taste to start working on you while we're eating. I'm supposed to drag everything out of you, so that's what I'll have to do, but I shouldn't start on it until the coffee, and by that time, if I'm any good, I'll have you in a frame of mind to let me even copy down your Social Security number."

"I would hate to miss that." She did try to smile. "It would be interesting to see you do it. But I promised my aunt I'd be back at the hotel by two-thirty—and by the way, I promised to bring you with me. Will you come?"

My brows went up. "To see Mrs. Boone?"

"Yes."

"She wants to see me?"

"Yes. Maybe only for fifteen minutes to discuss her looks. She didn't say."

"With girls over fifty, five is enough."

"She's not over fifty. She's forty-three."

"Five is still enough. But if we only have till two-thirty I'm afraid we'd better start without taking time to break down your resistance. How do you feel? Have you noticed any inclination to melt or relax or put your head on my shoulder?"

"Not the slightest." Her tone carried conviction. "The only impulse I've had was to pull your hair."

"Then it'll be a wonder," I said regretfully, "if you loosen up enough to tell me what size shoes you wear. However we'll see, as soon as he gets through serving. You haven't finished your cocktail."

She did so. The waiter gave us each a steaming plate of shrimps, cooked with cheese and covered with a spicy sauce, and individual bowls of salad on which he had just sprinkled a thin dressing. Nina speared a shrimp with her fork, decided it was too hot to go in whole, halved it, and conveyed a portion to her mouth. She was in no mood for tasting food, but she tasted that, and immediately got some more on her fork.

"I like this," she said. "Go on and drag things out of me."

I finished chewing my second shrimp and swallowed it. "My technique is a little unusual," I told her. "For instance, not only are all ten of you people being followed around, to see what you're up to now, but also your pasts are being drained through cheesecloth. How do you like this cheese?"

"I like it. I love it."

"Good. We'll come here often. There are probably a hundred men—no, more than that, I forgot how important this case is—investigating your people's pasts, to find out, for example, if Mrs. Boone was having secret trysts with Frank Thomas Erskine on the boardwalk at Atlantic City, or if you and Breslow are champing at the bit until he can get his wife to give him a divorce. That takes time and money, and my technique is different. I prefer to ask you and settle it. Are you?"

"Am I what? Champing?"

"At the bit."

"No. I'm champing shrimps."

I swallowed another one. "You see," I explained, "they're all up a stump, including Nero Wolfe. They're not trying to make it more complicated just for the hell of it. The most satisfactory way out of it, the way that would please nearly everybody most, including the investigators themselves, would be the simplest way, namely that one of those six NIA people killed Cheney Boone for the obvious motive, and then killed Phoebe Gunther for some related reason. But the trouble is that if that's how it was, how are you ever going to find out which one of the six did it, let alone prove it? Apparently not a chance in a billion. The New York police and the FBI have been working on it over a week now, giving it all they've got, and where are they? Tailing *you!*"

"Well." She herded cheese and sauce with her fork. "You're buying me a lunch."

"Certainly, and I'm telling you why, aside from your hair and other personal details. We're all sunk unless we can find a new angle. I came to you because there's a possibility that you know something about such an angle without realizing it. Naturally I'm assuming that you want the murderer found and punished. Otherwise—"

"I do. Of course I do."

"Then suppose we try the direct approach and see how it sounds. Did you know any of these NIA birds personally?"

"No."

"None of those six?"

"No."

"How about any NIA people at all? There were around fifteen hundred of them at that dinner."

"This seems perfectly silly."

"Then let's get it over with. Did you?"

"Maybe a few—or rather, their sons and daughters. I graduated from Smith a year ago, and you meet a lot of people. But if we went back over every minute of it, every word of every conversation, we wouldn't find anything remotely resembling an angle."

"You don't think it would do me any good to probe?"

"No." She glanced at her wrist watch. "Anyway, we haven't time."

"Okay. We can go back to it. How about your aunt? Those trysts with Erskine. Did she have trysts?"

Nina made a noise which, under the circumstances, was a fair substitute for a laugh. "Ask her. Maybe that's what she wants to see you about. If all the pasts are being investigated as you say they are, I should think it would be established by now that Aunt Luella was utterly and exclusively devoted to my uncle, and to everything he did and everything he stood for."

I shook my head. "You don't get it. That's just the point. To illustrate: what if Boone learned something in Washington that Tuesday afternoon about something Winterhoff had done, or something that made him decide to take a certain step affecting Winterhoff's line of business, and what if he told his wife about it when he saw her in their hotel room (which you might also have heard since you were there too), and what if Mrs. Boone happened to know Winterhoff, not for trysting purposes but just knew him, and what if later, in the reception room, she was talking with Winterhoff during her third cocktail, and what if unintentionally she gave him an idea of what was up? That's what I mean by a new angle. I could invent a thousand of them just as I invented that one, but what is needed is one that really happened. So I'm asking about your aunt's circle of acquaintance. Is that malevolent?"

She had been making steady progress with the shrimps, which had now cooled off enough to permit it. "No," she admitted, "but you'd better ask her. All I can tell you is about me."

"Sure. You're virtuous and noble. It shows in your chin. The herald angels sing. A in deportment."

"What do you want?" she demanded "Do you want me to tell you that I saw my aunt sneaking into a corner with Winterhoff or with any of those apes and whispering to him? Well, I didn't. And if I had—" She stopped.

"If you had would you tell me?"

"No. In spite of the fact that in my opinion my aunt is a pain in the neck."

"You don't like her?"

"No. I don't like her and I disapprove of her and I regard her as a grotesque relic. That's spread all over my past, but it's strictly personal."

"You don't go so far as to accept Breslow's suggestion that Mrs. Boone killed her husband on account of jealousy of Phoebe Gunther, and later, at Wolfe's house, finished up?"

"No, does anybody?"

"I couldn't say." Having disposed of the last shrimp, I started on the salad. "I don't. But it does seem to be a sound idea that Mrs. Boone was jealous of Phoebe Gunther."

"Certainly she was. There are several thousand girls and women working for the BPR, and she was jealous of all of them."

"Yeah. Chiefly on account of her nose, of course. But Phoebe Gunther wasn't just one of thousands. Wasn't she special?"

"She was indeed." Nina flashed me a quick glance which I failed to interpret. "She was extremely special."

"Was she going to do anything as trite as having a baby?"

"Oh, good lord." Nina pulled her salad over. "You pick up all the crumbs, don't you?"

"Was she?"

"No. And my aunt had just as little reason to be jealous of her as of anybody else. Her idea that my uncle had wolf in him was simply silly."

"How well did you know Miss Gunther?"

"I knew her pretty well. Not intimately."

"Did you like her?"

"I—yes, I guess I liked her. I certainly admired her. Of course I envied her. I would have liked to have her job, but I wasn't foolish enough to think I could fill it. I'm too young for one thing, but that's only part of it, she wasn't such a lot older than me. She did field work for a year or so and made the best record in the whole organization, and then she was brought to the main office and before long she was on the inside of everything. Usually when an organization like that gets a new Dircctor he does a great deal of shifting around, but when my uncle was appointed there wasn't any shifting of Phoebe except that she got a raise in pay. If she had been ten years older and a man she would have been made Director when my uncle—died."

"How old was she?"

"Twenty-seven."

"Did you know her before you went to work for the BPR?"

"No, but I met her the first day I went there, because my uncle asked her to keep an eye on me."

"Did she do so?"

"In a way she did, yes, as much as she had time for. She was very important and very busy. She had BPR fever."

"Yeah?" I stopped a forkload of salad on its way to my mouth. "Bad?"

"One of the most severe cases on record?"

"What were the main symptoms?"

"It varies with character and temperament. In its simplest form, a firm belief that whatever the BPR does is right. There are all kinds of complications, from bitter and undying hatred of the NIA to a messianic yen to educate the young, depending on whether you are primarily a do-gooder or a fighter."

"Have you got it?"

"Certainly I have, but not in its acute form. With me it

was mostly a personal matter. I was very fond of my uncle." Her chin threatened to get out of control for a moment, and she paused to attend to that and then explained, "I never had a father, to know him, and I loved Uncle Cheney. I don't really know an awful lot about it, but I loved my uncle."

"Which complications did Phoebe have?"

"All of them." The chin was all right again. "But she was a born fighter. I don't know how much the enemies of the BPR, for instance the heads of the NIA, really knew about the insides of it, but if their intelligence was any good they must have known about Phoebe. She was actually more dangerous to them than my uncle was. I've heard my uncle say that. A political shake-up might have got him out, but as long as she was there it wouldn't have mattered much."

"That's a big help," I grumbled, "I don't think. It gives precisely the same motive, to the same people, for her as for him. If you call that a new angle . . ."

"I don't call it anything. You asked me."

"So I did. How about dessert?"

"I don't think so."

"You'd better. You're going to have to help me out with your aunt maybe all afternoon, and that will take extra energy since you don't like her. A good number here is walnut pudding with cinnamon."

She conceded that it was a good idea and I passed it on to the waiter. While our table was being cleared and we were waiting for the pudding and coffee, we continued on the subject of Phoebe Gunther, with no revelations coming out of it, startling or otherwise. I introduced the detail of the missing tenth cylinder, and Nina snorted at the suggestion that Phoebe might have had concealed relations with some NIA individual and had ditched the cylinder because it implicated him or might have. I gave her that and asked how about the possibility that the cylinder implicated Solomon Dexter or Alger Kates. What was wrong with that?

With her spoon in her hand ready to start on the pudding, she shook her head positively. She said it was loony. To suppose that Dexter would have done anything to hurt Boone, thereby hurting the BPR also, was absurd. "Besides, he was in Washington. He didn't get to New York until late that night, when he was sent for. As for Mr. Kates, good heavens, look at him! He's just an adding machine!"

"He is in a pig's eye. He's sinister."

She gaped. "Alger Kates sinister!"

"Anyhow, mysterious. Down at Wolfe's house that evening Erskine accused him of killing your uncle because he wanted to marry you and your uncle opposed it, and Kates let it stand that he did want to marry you, along with two hundred other lovesick BPR's, and then later that same evening I learn that he already has a wife who is at present in Florida, A married adding machine does not covet another lovely maiden."

"Puh. He was merely being gallant or polite."

"An adding machine is not gallant. Another thing, where does the dough come from to send his wife to Florida at the present rates and keep her there until the end of March?"

"Really." Nina stopped eating pudding. "No matter what Nero Wolfe charges the NIA, you're certainly trying your best to earn it! You'd just love to clear them completely—and it looks as if you don't care how you do it! Perhaps Mrs. Kates won some money at a church bingo. You ought to check on that!"

I grinned at her. "When your face is flushed like that it makes me feel like refusing to take any part of my salary in NIA money. Some day I'll tell you how wrong you are to suspect us of wanting to frame one of your heroes like Dexter or Kates." I glanced at my wrist. "You just have time to finish your cigarette and coffee.—What is it, Carlos?"

"Telephone, Mr. Goodwin. The middle booth."

I had a notion to tell him to say I had gone, because I had a natural suspicion that it was the creature I had bribed with three nickels merely wanting to know how much longer we were going to be in there, but I thought better of it and excused myself, since there was one other person who knew where I was.

It proved to be the one other person.

"Goodwin talking."

"Archie. Get down here at once."

"What for?"

"Without delay!"

"But listen. We're just leaving, to see Mrs. Boone. I've got her to agree to see me. I'll put her through a—"

"I said get down here."

There was no use arguing. He sounded as if six tigers were crouching before him, lashing their tails, ready to spring. I went back to the table and told Nina that our afternoon was ruined.

28.

HAVING delivered Nina at the Waldorf entrance, with my pet bribee on our tail in a taxi, and having crowded the lights and the congested traffic down and across to West Thirty-fifth Street, I was relieved to see, as I reached my destination and braked to a stop at the curb, that the house wasn't on fire. There were only two foreign items visible: a police car parked smack in front of the address, and a man on the stoop. He was seated on the top step, hunched over, looking gloomy and obstinate.

This one I knew by name, one Quayle. He was on his feet by the time I had mounted the steps, and accosted me with what was meant to be cordiality.

"Hello, Goodwin! This is a piece of luck. Don't anybody ever answer the bell here when you're away? I'll just go in with you."

"Unexpected pleasure," I told him, and used my key, turned the knob, and pushed. The door opened two inches and stopped. The chain bolt was on, as it often was during my absence. My finger went to the button and executed my private ring. In a minute Fritz's step came down the hall and he spoke to me through the crack:

"Archie, that's a policeman. Mr. Wolfe doesn't—"

"Of course he doesn't. Take off the bolt. Then keep your eye on us. This officer eagerly performing his duty might lose his balance and fall down the stoop, and I may need you as a witness that I didn't push him. He must be twice my age."

"You witty son of a bitch," Quayle said sadly, and sat down on the step again. I entered, marched down the hall to the office, and saw Wolfe there alone behind his desk, sitting up straight as a ramrod, his lips pressed together in a thin straight line, his eyes wide open, his hands resting on the desk before him with the fingers curved ready for a throat.

His eyes darted at me. "What the devil took you so long?"

"Now just a minute," I soothed him. "Aware that you were having a fit, I made it as fast as I could in the traffic. Is it a pinch?"

"It is insufferable. Who is Inspector Ash?"

"Ash? You remember him. He was a captain under Cramer

from 1938 to '43. Now in charge of Homicide in Queens. Tall guy, face all bones, plastic eyes, very incorruptible and no sense of humor. Why, what has he done?"

"Is the car in good condition?"

"Certainly. Why?"

"I want you to drive me to Police Headquarters."

"My God." So it was something not only serious, but drastic. Leaving the house, getting in the car, incurring all the outdoor risks, visiting a policeman; and besides all that, which was unheard of, almost certainly standing up the orchids for the regular four o'clock date. I dropped onto a chair, speechless, and gawked at him.

"Luckily," Wolfe said, "when that man arrived the door was bolted. He told Fritz that he had come to take me to see Inspector Ash. When Fritz gave him the proper reply he displayed a warrant for me as a material witness regarding the murder of Miss Gunther. He pushed the warrant in through the crack in the door and Fritz pushed it out again and closed the door, and, through the glass panel, saw him walk toward the corner, presumably to telephone, since he left his car there in front of my house."

"That alone," I remarked, "leaving his car in front of your house, shows the kind of man he is. It's not even his car. It belongs to the city."

Wolfe didn't even hear me. "I called Inspector Cramer's office and was told he was not available. I finally succeeded in reaching some person who spoke in behalf of Inspector Ash, and was told that the man they had sent here had reported by telephone, and that unless I admitted him, accepted service of the warrant, and went with him, a search warrant would be sent without delay. I then, with great difficulty, got to the Police Commissioner. He has no guts. He tried to be evasive. He made what he called a concession, stating that I could come to his office instead of Inspector Ash's. I told him that only by using physical force could I be transported in any vehicle not driven by you, and he said they would wait for me until half-past three but no longer. An ultimatum with a time limit. He also said that Mr. Cramer has been removed from the Boone-Gunther case and relieved of his command and has been replaced by Inspector Ash. That's the situation. It is unacceptable."

I was staring incredulously. "Cramer got the boot?"

"So Mr. What's-his-name said."

"Who, Hombert? The Commissioner?"

"Yes. Confound it, must I repeat the whole thing for you?"

"For God's sake, don't. Try to relax. I'll be damned. They

got Cramer." I looked at the clock. "It's five past three, and that ultimatum has probably got narrow margins. You hold it a minute and try to think of something pleasant."

I went to the front and pulled the curtain aside for a look through the glass, and saw that Quayle had acquired a colleague. The pair were sitting on the stoop with their backs to me. I opened the door and inquired affably:

"What's the program now?"

Quayle twisted around. "We've got another paper. Which we'll show when the time comes. The kind of law that opens all doors from the mightiest to the humblest."

"To be shown when? Three-thirty?"

"Go suck a pickle."

"Aw, tell him," the colleague growled. "What do you expect to get out of it, fame?"

"He's witty," Quayle said petulantly. He twisted back to me. "At three-thirty we phone in again for the word."

"That's more like it," I declared approvingly. "And what happens if I emerge with a large object resembling Nero Wolfe and wedge him into my car and drive off? Do you flash your first paper and interfere?"

"No. We follow you if it's straight to Centre Street. If you try detouring by way of Yonkers that's different."

"Okay. I'm accepting your word of honor. If you forget what you said and try to grab him I'll complain to the Board of Health. He's sick."

"What with?"

"Sitzenlust. Chronic. The opposite of wanderlust. You wouldn't want to jeopardize a human life, would you?"

"Yes."

Satisfied, I closed the door and returned to the office and told Wolfe, "All set. In spite of our having outriders I'm game either for Centre Street or for a dash for Canada, however you feel. You can tell me after we're in the car."

He started to get erect, his lips compressed tighter than ever.

29.

"YOU are not an attorney," Inspector Ash declared in an insulting tone, though the statement was certainly not an insult in itself. "Nothing that has been said or written to you by anyone whatever has the status of a privileged communication."

It was not a convention as I had expected. Besides Wolfe and me the only ones present were Ash, Police Commissioner Hombert, and District Attorney Skinner, which left Hombert's spacious and well-furnished corner office looking practically uninhabited, even considering that Wolfe counted for three. At least he was not undergoing downright physical hardship, since there had been found available a chair large enough to accommodate his beam without excessive squeezing.

But he was conceding nothing. "That remark," he told Ash in his most objectionable tone, "is childish. Suppose I have been told something that I don't want you to know about. Would I admit the fact and then refuse to tell you about it on the ground that it was a privileged communication? Pfui! Suppose you kept after me. I would simply tell you a string of lies and then what?"

Ash was smiling. His plastic eyes had the effect of reflecting all the light that came at them from the four big windows, as if their surfaces could neither absorb light nor give it out.

"The trouble with you, Wolfe," he said curtly, "is that you've been spoiled by my predecessor, Inspector Cramer. He didn't know how to handle you. You had him buffaloed. With me in charge you'll see a big difference. A month from now or a year from now you may still have a license and you may not. It depends on how you behave." He tapped his chest with his forefinger. "You know me. You may remember how far you got with that Boeddiker case over in Queens."

"I never started. I quit. And your abominable handling gave the prosecutor insufficient evidence to convict a murderer whose guilt was manifest. Mr. Ash, you are both a numskull and a hooligan."

"So you're going to try it on me." Ash was still smiling. "Maybe I won't give you even a month. I don't see why—"

"That will do for that," Hombert broke in.

"Yes, sir," Ash said respectfully. "I only wanted—"

"I don't give a damn what you only wanted. We're in one hell of a fix, and that's all I'm interested in. If you want to ride Wolfe on this case go as far as you like, but save the rest till later. It was your idea that Wolfe was holding out and it was time to put the screws on him. Go ahead. I'm all for that."

"Yes, sir." Ash had quit smiling to look stern. "I only know this, that in every case I've ever heard of where Wolfe horned in and got within smelling distance of money he has always managed to get something that no one else gets, and he always hangs onto it until it suits his convenience to let go."

"You're quite correct, Inspector," District Attorney Skinner said dryly. "You might add that when he does let go the result is usually disastrous for some lawbreaker."

"Yes?" Ash demanded. "And is that a reason for letting him call the tune for the Police Department and your office?"

"I would like to ask," Wolfe put in, "if I was hauled down here to listen to a discussion of my own career and character. This babbling is frivolous."

Ash was getting stirred up. He glared. "You were hauled down here," he rasped, "to tell us what you know, and everything you know, about these crimes. You say I'm a numskull. I don't say you're a numskull, far from it, here's my opinion of you in one short sentence. I wouldn't be surprised if you know something that gives you a good clear idea of who it was that killed Cheney Boone and the Gunther woman."

"Certainly I do. So do you."

They made movements and noises. I grinned around at them, nonchalant, to convey the impression that there was nothing to get excited about, because I had the conviction that Wolfe was overplaying it beyond all reason just to get even with them and it might have undesirable consequences. His romantic nature often led him to excesses like that, and once he got started it was hard to stop him, the stopping being one of my functions. Before their exclamations and head-jerkings were finished I stepped in.

"He doesn't mean," I explained hastily, "that we've got the murderer down in our car. There are details to be attended to."

Hombert's and Skinner's movements had been limited to minor muscular reactions, but Ash had left his chair and strode masterfully to within two feet of Wolfe, where he stopped short to gaze down at him. He stood with his hands behind his back, which was effective in a way, but it would have been an improvement if he had remembered that in the classic Napoleon stance the arms are folded.

"You either mean it," he said like a menace, "or you don't. If it's a bluff you'll eat it. If it isn't, for once in your life you're going to be opened up." His bony head swiveled to Hombert. "Let me take him, sir. Here in your office it might be embarrassing."

"Imbecile," Wolfe muttered. "Hopeless imbecile." He applied the levers and got himself to his feet. "I had reluctantly accepted the necessity of a long and fruitless discussion of a singularly difficult problem, but this is farcical. Take me home, Archie."

"No you don't," Ash said, even more a menace. He reached and gripped Wolfe's arm. "You're under arrest, my man. This time you—"

I was aware that Wolfe could move without delay when he had to, and, knowing what his attitude was toward anybody's hand touching him, I had prepared myself for motion when I saw Ash grab his arm, but the speed and precision with which he slapped Ash on the side of his jaw were a real surprise, not only to me but to Ash himself. Ash didn't even know it was coming until it was there, a healthy open-palm smack with a satisfactory sound effect. Simultaneously Ash's eyes glittered and his left fist started, and I propelled myself up and forward. The emergency was too split-second to permit anything fancy, so I simply inserted myself in between, and Ash's left collided with my right shoulder before it had any momentum to speak of. With great presence of mind I didn't even bend an elbow, merely staying there as a barrier; but Wolfe, who claims constantly to detest a hubbub, said through his teeth:

"Hit him, Archie. Knock him down."

By that time Hombert was there and Skinner was hovering. Seeing that they were voting against bloodshed, and not caring to be tossed in the coop for manhandling an inspector, I backed away. Wolfe glared at me and said, still through his tooth:

"I am under arrest. You are not. Telephone Mr. Parker to arrange for bail immed—"

"Goodwin is staying right here." Ash's eyes were really nasty. I had never had an impulse to send him a birthday greeting card, but I was surprised to learn how mean he was. "Or rather you're both going with me—"

"Now listen." Skinner had his hands spread out patting air, like a pleader calming a mob. "This is ridiculous. We all want—"

"Am I under arrrest?"

"Oh, forget that! Technically, I suppose—"

"Then I am. You can all go to the devil." Wolfe went back to the big chair and sat down. "Mr. Goodwin will telephone our lawyer. If you want me out of here send for someone to carry me. If you want me to discuss anything with you, if you want a word out of me, vacate those warrants and get rid of Mr. Ash. He jars me."

"I'll take him," Ash snapped. "He struck an officer."

Skinner and Hombert looked at each other. Then they looked at Wolfe, then at me, and then at each other again. Skinner shook his head emphatically. Hombert regarded Wolfe once more and then turned his gaze on Ash.

"Inspector," he said, "I think you had better leave this to the District Attorney and me. You haven't been in charge of this case long enough to—uh—digest the situation, and while I consented to your proposal to get Wolfe down here, I doubt if you're sufficiently aware of—uh—all the aspects. I have described to you the sources of the strongest pressure to take Inspector Cramer off of the case, which meant also removing him from his command, and therefore it is worth considering that Wolfe's client is the National Industrial Association. Whether we want to consider it or not, we have to. You'd better return to your office, give the reports further study, and continue operations. Altogether, at this moment, there are nearly four hundred men working on this case. That's enough of a job for one man."

Ash's jaw was working and his eyes were still glittering. "It's up to you, sir," he said with an effort. "As I told you, and as you already knew, Wolfe has been getting away with murder for years. If you want him to get away with calling one of your subordinates an imbecile and physically assaulting him, in your own office . . ."

"At the moment I don't care a damn who gets away with what." Hombert was a little exasperated. "I care about just one thing, getting this case solved, and if that doesn't happen soon I may not have any subordinates. Get back on the job and phone me if there's anything new."

"Yes, sir." Ash crossed to Wolfe, who was seated, until their toes touched. "Some day," he promised, "I'll help you lose some weight." Then he strode out of the room.

I returned to my chair. Skinner had already returned to his. Hombert stood looking at the door that had closed behind the Inspector, ran his fingers through his hair, shook his head slowly a few times, moved to his own chair behind his desk, sat, and lifted a receiver from its cradle. In a moment he spoke into the transmitter:

"Bailey? Have that warrant for the arrest of Nero Wolfe as a material witness vacated. Right away. No, just cancel it. Send me—"

"*And* the search warrant," I put in.

"Also the search warrant for Nero Wolfe's house. No, cancel that too. Send the papers to me."

He hung up and turned to Wolfe. "All right, you got away with it. Now what do you know?"

Wolfe sighed deep. A casual glance at his bulk might have given the impression that he was placid again, but to my experienced eye, seeing that he was tapping the arm of his chair with his middle finger, it was evident that there was still plenty of turmoil.

"First," he muttered, "I would like to learn something. Why was Mr. Cramer demoted and disgraced?"

"He wasn't."

"Nonsense. Whatever you want to call it, why?"

"Officially, for a change of scene. Off the record, because he lost his head, considering who the people are that are involved, and took on a bigger load than the Department could handle. Whether you like it or not, there's such a thing as a sense of proportion. You cannot treat some people like a bunch of waterfront hoodlums."

"Who brought the pressure?"

"It came from everywhere. I've never seen anything like it. I'm giving no names. Anyhow, that wasn't the only reason. Cramer was muffing it. For the first time since I've known him he got tangled up. Here at a conference yesterday morning he couldn't even discuss the problem intelligently. He had got his mind fixed on one aspect of it, one little thing, and that was all he could think of or talk about—that missing cylinder, the tenth cylinder that may or may not have been in the leather case Boone gave to Miss Gunther just before he was murdered."

"Mr. Cramer was concentrating on that?"

"Yes. He had fifty men looking for it, and he wanted to assign another fifty to it."

"And that was one of your reasons for removing him?"

"Yes. Actually the main reason."

Wolfe grunted. "Hah. Then you're an imbecile too. I didn't know Mr. Cramer had it in him to see that. This doubles my admiration and respect for him. Finding that cylinder, if not our only chance, is beyond all comparison our best one. If it is never found the odds are big that we'll never get the murderer."

A loud disgusted snort came from Skinner. "That's you all right, Wolfe! I suspected it was only fireworks. You said you've already got him."

"I said nothing of the sort."

"You said you know who it is."

"No." Wolfe was truculent. Having been aroused to the point of committing assault and battery, he had by no means calmed down again. "I said I know something that gives me a good clear idea of the murderer's identity, and I also said that you people know it too. You know many things that I don't know. Don't try to pretend that I bulldozed you into ejecting Mr. Ash and releasing me from custody by conveying the impression that I am prepared to name the culprit and supply the evidence. I am not."

Hombert and Skinner looked at each other. There was a silence.

"You impervious bastard," Skinner said, but wasting no energy on it.

"In effect, then," Hombert said resentfully, "you are saying that you have nothing to tell us, that you have nothing to offer, that you can't help us any."

"I'm helping all I can. I am paying a man twenty dollars a day to explore the possibility that Miss Gunther broke that cylinder into little pieces and put it in the rubbish receptacle in her apartment in Washington. That's going to an extreme, because I doubt if she destroyed it. I think she expected to use it some day."

Hombert shifted impatiently in his chair as if the idea of hunting for a lousy cylinder, possibly broken anyhow, only irritated him. "Suppose," he said, "you tell us what it is we all know that gives you a good clear idea of who the murderer is, including the who. Off the record."

"It isn't any one thing."

"I don't care if it's a dozen things. I'll try to remember them. What are they?"

Wolfe shook his head. "No, sir."

"Why not?"

"Because of your idiotic treatment of Mr. Cramer. If it seemed to make sense to you, and I believe it would, you would pass it on to Mr. Ash, and heaven knows what he would do. He might even, by pure chance, do something that would result in his solving the case, and I would stop short of nothing to prevent that outcome." Wolfe's middle finger started tapping again. "Help Mr. Ash to a triumph? God forbid!" He frowned at Hombert. "Besides, I've already given you the best advice I've got. Find that cylinder. Put a hundred men on it, a thousand. Find it!"

"We're not neglecting the damn cylinder. How about this, do you think Miss Gunther knew who killed Boone?"

"Certainly she did."

Skinner broke in. "Naturally you'd like that," he said pessimistically, "since it would eliminate your clients. If Miss Gunther knew who it was, and it was an NIA man, she would have handed it to us on a platter. So if she did know, it was and is one of the other four—Dexter or Kates or one of the Boone women."

"Not at all," Wolfe contradicted him.

"But damn it, of course!"

"No." Wolfe sighed. "You're missing the whole point. What has been the outstanding fact about this case for a whole week now? What was its peculiar characteristic? This, that the public, the people, had immediately brought the case to trial as usual, without even waiting for an arrest, and instead of the customary prolonged disagreement and dissension regarding various suspects, they reached an immediate verdict. Almost unanimously they convicted—this was the peculiar fact—not an individual, but an organization. The verdict was that the National Industrial Association had murdered Cheney Boone. Now what if you were Miss Gunther and knew who had killed Boone? No matter how you knew, that's another question; the point is that you knew. I think she did know. Let's suppose she knew it was young Mr. Erskine. Would she have exposed him? No. She was devoted to the interests of her own organization, the BPR. She saw the rising tide of resentment and indignation against the NIA, constantly increasing in force and intensity. She saw that it might result, if sustained long enough, in completely discrediting the NIA and its purposes, policies, and objectives. She was intelligent enough to calculate that if an individual, no matter who, were arrested for the murder with good evidence, most of the resentment against the NIA would be diverted away from it as an organization."

Wolfe sighed again. "What would she do? If she had evidence that pointed to Mr. Erskine, or to anyone else, she would suppress it; but she wouldn't destroy it, for she wouldn't want the murderer eventually to escape his punishment. She would put it where it wouldn't be found, but where she could retrieve it and produce it when the time came, when the NIA had been sufficiently damaged. It is not even necessary to assume loyalty to the BPR as her dominating motive. Suppose it was personal devotion to Mr. Boone and a desire to avenge him. The best possible revenge, the perfect revenge, would be to use his death and the manner of it for the discomfiture and the destruction of the organization which had hated him and tried to thwart him. In my opinion Miss Gunther was capable of that. She was a remarkable young woman. But she made the mistake of permitting the murderer to learn that she knew who he was, how is still another question, and that she paid for."

Wolfe raised his hand and let if fall. "However, note this. Her own death served her purpose too. In the past two days the wave of anger against the NIA has increased tremendously. It is going deep into the feeling of the people, and soon it will be impossible to dredge it out again. She was a remarkable woman. No, Mr. Skinner, Miss Gunther's knowing the identity of the murderer would not eliminate my clients. Besides, no man is my client, and no men are. My checks come from the National Industrial Association, which, having no soul, could not possibly commit a murder."

Wolfe cocked an eye at Hombert. "Speaking of checks. You have seen the NIA advertisement offering a reward of one hundred thousand dollars. You might let your men know that whoever finds the missing cylinder will get that reward."

"Yes?" Hombert was skeptical. "You're as bad as Cramer. What makes you so damn sure about that cylinder? Have you got it in your pocket?"

"No. If I had!"

"What makes you so sure about it?"

"Well. I can't put it in a sentence."

"We've got all the time there is."

"Didn't Mr. Cramer explain it to you?"

"Forget Cramer. He's out of it."

"Which is nothing to your credit, sir." Wolfe rearranged his pressures and angles, shifting the mass to get the center of gravity exactly right for maximum comfort. An unaccustumed chair always presented him with a complicated engineering problem. "You really want me to go into this?"

"Yes."

"Mr. Skinner?"

"Yes."

"All right, I will." Wolfe closed his eyes. "It was apparent from the beginning that Miss Gunther was lying about the leather case. Mr. Cramer knew that, of course. Four people stated that they saw her leaving the reception room with it, people who couldn't possibly have been aware, at the time, that its contents had anything to do with the murder—unless they were all involved in a murder conspiracy, which is preposterous—and therefore had no valid reason for mendacity. Also, Mrs. Boone was barely able to stop herself short of accusing Miss Gunther of falsehood, and Mrs. Boone was at the same table with her in the ballroom. So Miss Gunther was lying. You see that."

"Keep right on," Skinner growled.

"I intend to. Why did she lie about the case and pretend that it had disappeared? Obviously because she didn't want the text of the cylinders, one or more of them, to become known. Why didn't she? Not merely because it contained confidential BPR information or intent. Such a text, as she knew, could safely have been entrusted to FBI ears, but she audaciously and jauntily suppressed it. She did that because something in it pointed definitely and unmistakably to the murderer of Mr. Boone. She—"

"No," Hombert objected. "That's out. She lied about the case before she could have known that. She told us Wednesday morning, the morning after Boone was killed, about leaving the case on the window sill in the reception room, before she had had an opportunity to listen to what was on the cylinders. So she couldn't have known that."

"Yes she could."

"She could tell what was on those cylinders without having access to a Stenophone machine?"

"Certainly. At least one of them. Mr. Boone told her what was on it when he gave her the leather case Tuesday evening, in the room there where he was soon to die. She lied about that too; naturally she had to. She lied about it to me, most convincingly, in my office Friday evening. I should have warned her then that she was being foolhardy to the point of imprudence, but I didn't. I would have wasted my breath. Caution with respect to personal peril was not in her makeup—as the event proved. If it had been, she would not have permitted a man whom she knew to be capable of murder get close to her, alone, on the stoop of my house."

Wolfe shook his head, his eyes still closed. "She was really extraordinary. It would be interesting to know where she concealed the case, containing the cylinders, up to Thursday afternoon. It would have been too risky to hide it in Mr. Kates's apartment, which might have been searched by the police at any moment. Possibly she checked it in the Grand Central parcel room, though that seems a little banal for her. At any rate, she had it with her in her suitcase when she went to Washington Thursday afternoon, with Mr. Dexter and with your permission."

"Cramer's permission," Hombert grumbled.

Wolfe ignored it. "I would like to emphasize," he said with his voice up a little, "that none of this is conjecture except unimportant details of chronology and method. In Washington Miss Gunther went to her office, listened to the cylinders, and learned which one bore the message that Mr. Boone had told her about. Doubtless she wanted to know exactly what it said, but also she wanted to simplify her problem. It isn't easy to conceal an object the size of that case from an army of expert searchers. She wanted to reduce it to one little cylinder. Another thing, she had contrived a plot. She took the nine eliminated cylinders to her Washington apartment and hid them casually in a hatbox on a closet shelf. She also took ten other cylinders that had been previously used which were there in her office, put them in the leather case, brought it with her when she returned to New York, and checked it in the Grand Central parcel room.

"That was in preparation for her plot, and she probably would have proceeded with it the next day, using the police for the mystification, if it hadn't been for that invitation I sent around for a discussion at my office. She decided to wait for developments. Why she ignored my invitation I don't know, and I shall intrude no guesses. That same evening, Friday, Mr. Goodwin went after her and brought her to my office. She had made a profound impression on him, and she struck me as being of uncommon quality. Evidently her opinion of us was less flattering. She formed the idea that we were more vulnerable to guile than the police; and the next day, Saturday, after she had mailed the parcel room check to Mr. O'Neill and made the phone call to him, giving the name of Dorothy Unger, she sent me a telegram, signing Mr. Breslow's name to it, conveying the notion that observation of Mr. O'Neill's movements might be profitable. We validated her appraisal of us. Mr. Goodwin was at Mr. O'Neill's address bright and early Sunday morning, as Miss Gunther intended him to be. When Mr. O'Neill emerged he was followed, and you know what happened."

"I don't understand," Skinner interposed, "why O'Neill was such an easy sucker for that Dorothy Unger phone call. Didn't the damn fool suspect a plant? Or is he a damn fool or something else?"

Wolfe shook his head. "Now you're asking for more than I've got. Mr. O'Neill is a headstrong and bumptious man, which may account for it; and we know that he was irresistibly tempted to learn what was on those cylinders, whether because he had killed Mr. Boone or for some other reason is yet to be discovered. Presumably Miss Gunther knew what might be expected of him. Anyhow her plot was moderately successful. It kept us all in that side alley for a day or two, it further jumbled the matter of the cylinders and the leather case, and it was one more involvement of an NIA man, without, however, the undesirable result—undesirable for Miss Gunther—of exposing him as the murderer. She was saving that—the disclosure of the murderer's identity and the evidence she had—for the time that would best suit her purpose."

"You've got pictures of all this," Skinner said sarcastically. "Why didn't you call her on the phone or get her in your office and lecture her on the duties of a citizen?"

"It was impractical. She was dead."

"Oh? Then you didn't know it all until after she had been killed?"

"Certainly not. How the devil could I? Some of it, yes, it doesn't matter how much. But when word came from Washington that they had found in Miss Gunther's apartment, perfunctorily concealed, nine of the cylinders Mr. Boone had dictated the afternoon of his death—nine, not ten—there was the whole story. There was no other acceptable explanation. All questions became paltry and pointless except the one question: where is the tenth cylinder?"

"Wherever you start a sentence," Hombert complained grouchily, "it always ends on that goddam cylinder!"

Wolfe opened his eyes enough to pick Hombert out. "You try doing a sentence that makes any sense and leave the cylinder out."

Skinner demanded, "What if she threw it in thc river?"

"She didn't."

"Why not?"

"I've already told you. Because she intended to use it, when the time came, to get the murderer punished."

"What if you're making your first and only mistake and she *did* throw it in the river?"

"Drag the river. All the rivers she could reach."

"Don't be whimsical. Answer my question."

Wolfe's shoulders went perceptibly up and down. "In that case we would be licked. We'd never get him."

"I think," Hombert said pointedly, "that it is conceivable that you would like to sell a bill of goods. I don't say you're a barefaced liar."

"I don't say I'm not, Mr. Hombert. We all take those chances when we exchange words with other people. So I might as well go home—"

"Wait a minute," Skinner snapped. "Do you mean that as an expert investigator you advise abandoning all lines of inquiry except the search for that cylinder?"

"I shouldn't think so." Wolfe frowned, considering. "Especially not with a thousand men or more at your disposal. Of course I don't know what has been done and what hasn't, but I know how such things go and I doubt if much has been overlooked in a case of this importance, knowing Mr. Cramer as I do. For instance, that piece of iron pipe; I suppose every possible effort has been made to discover where it came from. The matter of arrivals at my house Monday evening has of course been explored with every resource and ingenuity. The tenants of all the buildings in my block on both sides of the street have naturally been interviewed, on the slim chance, unlikely in that quiet neighborhood, that somebody saw or heard something. The question of opportunity alone, the evening of the dinner at the Waldorf, must have kept a dozen men busy for a week, and perhaps you're still working on it. Inquiries regarding relationships, both open and concealed, the checking and rechecking of Mr. Dexter's alibi—these and a thousand other details have unquestionably been competently and thoroughly attended to."

Wolfe wiggled a finger. "And where are you? So sunk in a bog of futility and bewilderment that you resort to such monkey tricks as ditching Mr. Cramer, replacing him with a buffoon like Mr. Ash, and swearing out a warrant for my arrest! Over a long period I have become familiar with the abilities and performances of the New York police, and I never expected to see the day when the inspector heading the Homicide Squad would try to solve a difficult murder case by dragging me off to a cell, attacking my person, putting me in handcuffs, and threatening me with mayhem!"

"That's a slight exaggeration. This is not a cell, and I don't—"

"He intended to," Wolfe asserted grimly. "He would have. Very well. You have asked my advice. I would continue, within reason, all lines of inquiry that have already been started, and initiate any others that offer any promise whatever, because no matter what the cylinder gives you—if and when you find it—you will almost certainly need all available scraps of support and corroboration. But the main chance, the only real hope, is the cylinder. I suggest you try this. You both met Miss Gunther? Good. Sit down and shut your eyes and imagine it is last Thursday afternoon, and you are Miss Gunther, sitting in your office in the BPR headquarters in Washington. You have decided what you are going to do with the leather case and the nine eliminated cylinders; forget all that. In your hand is *the* cylinder, and the question is what to do with it. Here's what you're after: you want to preserve it against any risk of damage, you want it easily accessible should you need it on short notice, and you want to be certain that no matter how many people look for it, or who, with whatever persistence and ingenuity, it will not be found."

Wolfe looked from one to the other. "There's your little problem, Miss Gunther. Anything so simple, for example, as concealing it there in the BPR office is not even to be considered. Something far above that, something really fine, must be conceived. Your own apartment would be merely ridiculous; you show that you are quite aware of that by disposing of the other nine cylinders as you do. Perhaps the apartment of a friend or colleague you can trust? This is murder; this is of the utmost gravity and of ultimate importance; would you trust any other human being that far? You are ready now to leave, to go to your apartment first and then take a plane to New York. You will probably be in New York some days. Do you take the cylinder with you or leave it in Washington? If so, where? Where? Where?"

Wolfe flipped a hand. "There's your question, gentlemen.

Answer it the way Miss Gunther finally answered it, and your worries are ended." He stood up. "I am spending a thousand dollars a day trying to learn how Miss Gunther answered it." He was multiplying by two and it wasn't his money he was spending, but at least it wasn't a barefaced lie. "Come, Archie. I want to go home."

They didn't want him to go, even then, which was the best demonstration to date of the pitiable condition they were in. They certainly were stymied, flummoxed, and stripped to the bone. Wolfe magnanimously accommodated them by composing a few more well-constructed sentences, properly furnished with subjects, predicates, and subordinate clauses, none of which meant a damn thing, and then marched from the room with me bringing up the rear. He had postponed his exit, I noticed, until after a clerk had entered to deliver some papers to Hombert's desk, which had occurred just as Wolfe was telling the P.C. and D.A. to shut their eyes and pretend they were Miss Gunther.

Driving back home he sat in the back seat, as usual, clutching the toggle, because of his theory that when—not if and when, just when—the car took a whim to dart aside and smash into some immovable object, your chances in back, hopeless as they were, were slightly better than in front. On the way down to Centre Street I had, on request, given him a sketch of my session with Nina Boone, and now, going home, I filled in the gaps. I couldn't tell whether it contained any morsel that he considered nutritious, because my back was to him and his face wasn't in my line of vision in the mirror, and also because the emotions that being in a moving vehicle aroused in him were too overwhelming to leave any room for minor reactions.

As Fritz let us in and we entered the hall and I attended to hat and coat disposal, Wolfe looked almost good-humored. He had beaten a rap and was home safe, and it was only six o'clock, time for beer. But Fritz spoiled it at once by telling us that we had a visitor waiting in the office. Wolfe scowled at him and demanded in a ferocious whisper:

"Who is it?"

"Mrs. Cheney Boone."

"Good heavens. That hysterical gammer?"

Which was absolutely unfair. Mrs. Boone had been in the house just twice, both times under anything but tranquil circumstances, and I hadn't seen the faintest indication of hysteria.

30.

I HAD made a close and prolonged study of Wolfe's attitude toward women. The basic fact about a woman that seemed to irritate him was that she was a woman; the long record showed not a single exception; but from there on the documentation was cockeyed. If woman as woman grated on him you would suppose that the most womany details would be the worst for him, but time and again I have known him to have a chair placed for a female so that his desk would not obstruct his view of her legs, and the answer can't be that his interest is professional and he reads character from legs, because the older and dumpier she is the less he cares where she sits. It is a very complex question and some day I'm going to take a whole chapter for it. Another little detail: he is much more sensitive to women's noses than he is to men's. I have never been able to detect that extremes or unorthodoxies in men's noses have any effect on him, but in women's they do. Above all he doesn't like a pug, or in fact a pronounced incurve anywhere along the bridge.

Mrs. Boone had a pug, and it was much too small for the surroundings. I saw him looking at it as he leaned back in his chair. So he told her in a gruff and inhospitable tone, barely not boorish:

"I have ten minutes to spare, madam."

Entirely aside from the nose she looked terrible. She had had a go at her compact, but apparently with complete indifference to the result, and anyway it would have been a job for a make-up artist. She was simply all shot and her face had quit trying to do any pretending about it.

"Naturally," she said, in a voice that was holding up much better than the face, "you're wondering why I'm here."

"Naturally," Wolfe agreed.

"I mean why I came to see you, since you're on the other side. It's because I phoned my cousin this morning and he told me about you."

"I am not," Wolfe said curtly, "on the other side or any side. I have undertaken to catch a murderer. Do I know your cousin?"

She nodded. "General Carpenter. That was my maiden name. He is my first cousin. He's in a hospital after an operation, or he would have come to help me when my husband was killed. He told me not to believe anything you said but to do whatever you told me to do. He said that you have your own private set of rules, and that if you are working on a case of murder the only one that can really rely on you is the murderer. Since you know my cousin, you know what he meant. I'm used to him."

She stopped, looked at me and back at Wolfe, and used her handkerchief on her lower lip and at the corners, which didn't improve things any. When her hand went back to her lap it was gripping the handkerchief as if it was afraid that someone was planning to snatch it.

"And?" Wolfe prompted her.

"So I came to see you to get some advice. Or maybe I ought to say make up my mind whether I want to ask your advice. I have to get some from somebody, and I don't know—" She looked at me again, returned to Wolfe, and made a gesture with the hand that wasn't guarding the handkerchief. "Do I have to tell you why I prefer not to go to someone in the FBI or the police?"

"You are under no compulsion, madam, to tell me anything at all. You've already been talking three or four minutes."

"I know. My cousin warned me that you would be incredibly rude. —Then I might as well come right out and say that I think I am responsible for the death of Phoebe Gunther."

"That's an uncomfortable thought," muttered Wolfe. "Where did you get it?"

"That's what I want to tell you, and I suppose I'm really going to or I wouldn't have come here, but while I was sitting here waiting I got up to leave a dozen times and then sat down again. I don't know what to do and last night I thought I was going crazy. I always depended on my husband to make important decisions. I don't want to tell the police or the FBI because I may have committed some kind of a crime, I don't know. But it seems silly to tell you on account of the way my husband felt about the NIA, and of course I feel the same way about them, and you're working for them, you're on their side. I suppose I ought to go to a lawyer, and I know lots of lawyers, but there doesn't seem to be one I could tell this to. They all seem to do all the talking and I never understand what they're saying."

That should have softened Wolfe up. He did get a little more receptive, taking the trouble to repeat that he wasn't on any side. "For me," he stated, "this is not a private feud, whatever it may be for others. What was the crime you committed?"

"I don't know—if it was one."

"What did you do?"

"I didn't do anything. That's the trouble. What happened was that Miss Gunther told me what she was doing and I promised her I wouldn't tell anyone and I didn't, and I have a feeling—"

She stopped. In a moment she went on, "That isn't true, I haven't just got a feeling. I'm sure."

"Sure of what?"

"I'm sure that if I had told the police what she told me she wouldn't have been killed. But I didn't tell, because she explained that what she was doing was helping the BPR and hurting the NIA, and that was what my husband would have wanted more than anything else." The widow was staring at Wolfe's face as if she were trying to see inside. "And she was perfectly correct. I'm still making up my mind whether to tell you about it. In spite of what you say, there's my husband's side and there's the other side, and you're working for the NIA. After I talked with my cousin I thought I'd come and see what you sounded like."

"What do I sound like?"

"I don't know." Her hand fluttered vaguely. "I really don't know."

Wolfe frowned at her in silence, then heaved a sigh and turned to me.

"Archie."

"Yes, sir?"

"Your notebook. Take a letter. To be mailed this evening so it will be delivered in the morning. To the National Industrial Association, attention Mr. Frank Thomas Erskine.

"Gentlemen: The course events have taken obliges me to inform you that it will be impossible for me to continue to act in your behalf with regard to the investigation of the murders of Mr. Cheney Boone and Miss Phoebe Gunther. Therefore I enclose herewith my check for thirty thousand dollars, returning the retainer you have paid me and ending my association with you in this matter. Sincerely."

I made the last scratch and looked at him. "Do I draw the check?"

"Certainly. You can't enclose it if it hasn't been drawn." Wolfe's eyes moved to the visitor. "There, Mrs. Boone, that should have some effect on your reluctance. Even accepting your point of view, that I was on the other side, now I am not. What did Miss Gunther tell you she was doing?"

The widow was gazing at him. "Thirty thousand dollars?" she asked incredulously.

"Yes." Wolfe was smirking. "A substantial sum."

"But was that all the NIA was paying you? Just *thirty thousand?* I supposed it was twenty times that! They have hundreds of millions—billions!"

"It was only the retainer," Wolfe said testily. The smirk was gone. "Anyway, I am now a neutral. What did Miss Gunther tell you?"

"But now—but now you're not getting anything at all!" Mrs. Boone was utterly bewildered. "My cousin told me that during the war you worked hard for the government for nothing, but that you charge private people outrageous prices. I ought to tell you—if you don't know—that I can't afford to pay you anything outrageous. I could—" she hesitated. "I could give you a check for a hundred dollars."

"I don't want a check." Wolfe was exasperated. "If I can't have a client in this case without being accused of taking sides in a sanguinary vendetta, I don't want a client. Confound it, what did Miss Gunther tell you?"

Mrs. Boone looked at me, and I had the uncomfortable feeling that she was trying to find some sort of resemblance to her dead husband, he being gone and therefore no longer available for important decisions. I thought it might possibly help if I nodded at her reassuringly, so I did. Whether that broke the tie or not I don't know, but something did, for she spoke to Wolfe:

"She knew who killed my husband. My husband told her something that day when he gave her the leather case, and she knew from that, and also he had dictated something on one of those cylinders that told about it, so the cylinder was evidence, and she had it. She was keeping it and she intended to give it to the police, but she was waiting until the talk and the rumors and the public feeling had done as much damage as possible to the NIA. She told me about it because I went to her and told her I knew she wasn't telling the truth about that leather case, I knew she had had it with her at the table in the dining room, and I wasn't going to keep still about it any longer. She told me what she was doing so I wouldn't tell the police about the case."

"When was that? What day?"

She thought a moment, the crease deepening in her forehead, and then shook her head uncertainly. "The days," she said. "The days are all mixed up."

"Of course they are, Mrs. Boone. It was Friday evening when you were here with the others the first time, when you almost spoke up about it and changed your mind. Was it before that, or after?"

"It was after. It was the next day."

"Then it was Saturday. Another thing that will help you to place it, Saturday morning you received an envelope in the mail containing your wedding picture and automobile license. Do you remember that? It was the same day?"

She nodded with assurance. "Yes, of course it was. Because I spoke of that, and she said she had written a letter to him—to the man who killed my husband—she knew my husband had always carried the wedding picture in the wallet that was missing—he had carried it for over twenty years—twenty-three years—"

The widow's voice got away from her. She gave it up and gulped, sat without trying to go on, and gulped again. If she lost control completely and started noises and tears there was no telling what Wolfe would do. He might even have tried to act human, which would have been an awful strain on all of us. So I told her gruffly:

"Okay, Mrs. Boone, take your time. Whenever you get ready, what did she write a letter to the murderer for? To tell him to send you the wedding picture?"

She nodded and got enough voice back to mumble, "Yes."

"Indeed," Wolfe said to help out.

The widow nodded again. "She told me that she knew I would want that picture, and she wrote him to say that she knew about him and he must send it to me."

"What else did she write him?"

"I don't know. That's all she told me about it."

"But she told you who he was."

"No, she didn't." Mrs. Boone halted again for a moment, still getting her voice back into place. "She said she wouldn't tell me that, because it would be too much to expect me not to show that I knew. She said I didn't need to worry about his not being punished, there would be no doubt about that, and besides it would be dangerous for me to know. That's where I now think I did wrong—that's why I said I'm responsible for her death. If it would have been dangerous for me it was dangerous for her, especially after she wrote him that letter. I should have made her tell the police about it, and if she wouldn't do it I should have broken my promise to her and told the police myself. Then she wouldn't have been killed. Anyway she said she thought she was breaking a law, withholding information and concealing evidence, so I have that on my mind too, helping her break a law."

"You can stop worrying about that, at least," Wolfe assured her. "I mean the lawbreaking. That part of it's all right. Or it will be, as soon as you tell me, and I tell the police, where Miss Gunther put the cylinder."

"But I can't. That's another thing. I don't know. She didn't tell me."

Wolfe's eyes had popped wide open. "Nonsense!" he said rudely. "Of course she told you!"

"She did not. That's one reason I came to see you. She said I didn't need to worry about the man who killed my husband being punished. But if that's the only evidence . . ."

Wolfe's cyes had gone shut again. There was a long silence. Mrs. Boone looked at me, possibly still in search of a resemblance, but whatever she was looking for her expression gave no indication that she was finding it. Finally she spoke to Wolfe again:

"So you see why I need advice . . ."

His lids went up enough to make slits. In his place I would at least have been grateful for all the corroboration of the guesses I had made, but apparently he was too overcome by his failure to learn where the cylinder was.

"I regret, madam," he said, without any noticeable tremor of regret or anything like it, "that I can't be of any help to you. There is nothing I can do. All I can give you is what you said you came for, advice, and you are welcome to that. Mr. Goodwin will drive you back to your hotel. Arriving therc, telephone the police immediately that you have information for them. When they come, tell them everything you have told me, and answer their questions as long as you can stand it. You need have no fear of being regarded as guilty of lawbreaking. I agree with you that if you had broken your promise to Miss Gunther she would probably not have been killed, but it was she who asked you for the promise, so the responsibility is hers. Besides, she can afford it; it is astonishing, the burden of responsibility that dead people can bear up under. Dismiss that from your mind too if you can." He was on his feet. "Good afternoon, madam."

So I did get to drive a female Boone home from our office, though not Nina. Since it appeared that she had given us all she had and was therefore of no further immediate interest, I didn't even bother to discover whether anyone was on her tail and confined myself to the duties of a chauffeur. She didn't seem to care about conversing, which simplified matters. I delivered her safely at the Waldorf entrance and headed back downtown. Aside from the attention to driving, which was automatic, there was no point in trying to put my mind on my work, since I was being left out in the cold and therefore had no work, so I let it drift to Phoebe Gunther. I went back to the times I had been with her, how she had talked and acted, with my present knowledge of what she had been doing, and decided she had been utterly all right. I have an inclination to pick flaws, especially where young women are concerned, but on this occasion I didn't have the list started by the time I got back home.

Wolfe was drinking beer, as I observed when I stepped inside the office door merely to tell him:

"I'll be upstairs. I always like to wash my hands after I've been with certain kinds of policemen, meaning Inspector Ash, and I've—"

"Come in here. That letter and check. We'd better get that done."

I gawked. "What, to the NIA?"

"Yes."

"My God, you don't mean you're actually going to send it?"

"Certainly. Didn't I tell that woman I would? Wasn't it with that understanding that she told me things?"

I sat down at my desk and regarded him piercingly. "This," I said sternly, "is not being eccentric. This is plain loony. What about Operation Payroll? And where did you suddenly get a scruple? And anyway, she didn't tell you the one thing you wanted to know." I abruptly got respectful. "I regret to report, sir, that the checkbook is lost."

He grunted. "Draw the check and type the letter. At once." He pointed to a stack of envelopes on his desk. "Then you can go through these reports from Mr. Bascom's office. They just came by messenger."

"But with no client—shall I phone Bascom to call it off?"

"Certainly not."

I went to the safe for the checkbook. As I filled out the stub I remarked, "Statistics show that forty-two and three-tenths per cent of all geniuses go crazy sooner or later."

He had no comment. He merely drank beer and sat. Now that I was to be permitted to know what Bascom's men were doing, he wouldn't even co-operate enough to slit open the envelopes. Whatever it was it must be good, since he evidently intended to go on paying for it with his own dough. I pounded the typewriter keys in a daze. When I put the check and letter before him to be signed I said plaintively:

"Excuse me for mentioning it, but a century from Mrs. Boone would have helped. That seems to be more our speed. She said she could afford it."

He used the blotter. "You'd better take this to the post office. I suspect the evening collection from that box doesn't get made sometimes."

So I had some more chauffeuring to do. It was only a ten-minute walk to the post office on Ninth Avenue and back, but I was in no mood for walking. I only like to walk when I can see some future ahead of me. Returning, I put the car in the garage, since the evening would obviously be a complete blank.

Wolfe was still in the office, outwardly perfectly normal. He glanced at me, then at the clock, and back at me.

"Sit down a moment, Archie. You'll have plenty of time to wash before dinner. Dr. Vollmer is coming to see us later, and you need some instructions."

At least his mind was still functioning enough to send for a doctor.

31.

DOC VOLLMER was due to arrive at ten o'clock. At five minutes to ten the stage was set, up in Wolfe's bedroom. I was in Wolfe's own chair by the reading lamp, with a magazine. Wolfe was in bed. Wolfe in bed was always a remarkable sight, accustomed to it as I was. First the low footboard, of streaky anselmo—yellowish with sweeping dark brown streaks—then the black silk coverlet, next the wide expanse of yellow pajama top, and last the flesh of the face. In my opinion Wolfe was quite aware that black and yellow are a flashy combination, and he used it deliberately just to prove that no matter how showy the scene was he could dominate it. I have often thought that I would like to see him try it with pink and green. The rest of the room—rugs and furniture and curtains—was okay, big and comfortable and all right to be in.

Doc Vollmer, admitted downstairs by Fritz and knowing his way around the house, came up the one flight alone and walked into the room, the door standing open. He was carrying his toolbox. He had a round face and round ears, and two or three years had passed since he had given up any attempt to stand with his belly in and his chest out. I told him hello and shook hands, and then he went to the bedside with a friendly greeting and his hand extended.

Wolfe twisted his neck to peer at the offered hand, grunted skeptically, and muttered, "No, thank you. What's the ceiling on it? I don't want any."

Standing at the footboard, I began hastily, "I should have explained—" but Wolfe broke in, thundering at Vollmer,

"Do you want to pay two dollars a pound for butter? Fifty cents for shoestrings? A dollar for a bottle of beer? Twenty dollars for one orchid, one ordinary half-wilted Laeliocattleya? Well, confound it, answer me!" Then he quit thundering and started muttering.

Vollmer lowered himself to the edge of a chair, put his toolbox on the floor, blinked several times at Wolfe, and then at me.

I said, "I don't know whether it's the willies or what."

Wolfe said, "You accuse me of getting you here under false pretenses. You accuse me of wanting to borrow money from you. Just because I ask you to lend me five dollars until the beginning of the next war, you accuse me!" He shook a warning finger in the direction of Vollmer's round astonished face. "Let me tell you, sir, you will be next! I admit that I am finished; I am finally driven to this extremity. They have done for me; they have broken me; they are still after me." His voice rose to thunder again. "And you, you incomparable fool, you think to escape! Archie tells me you are masquerading as a doctor. Bah! They'll take your clothes off! They'll examine every inch of your skin, as they did mine! They'll find the mark!" He let his head fall back on the pillow, closed his eyes, and resumed muttering.

Vollmer looked at me with a gleam in his eyes and inquired, "Who wrote his script for him?"

Managing somehow to control the muscles around my mouth, I shook my head despairingly. "He's been like this for several hours, ever since I brought him back home."

"Oh, he's been out of the house?"

"Yes. From three-fifteen till six o'clock. Under arrest."

Vollmer turned to Wolfe. "Well," he said decisively. "The first thing is to get some nurses. Where's the phone? Either that or take him to a hospital."

"That's the ticket," I agreed. "It's urgent. We must act."

Wolfe's eyes came open. "Nurses?" he asked contemptuously. "Pfui. Aren't you a physician? Don't you know a nervous breakdown when you see one?"

"Yes," Vollmer said emphatically.

"What's the matter with it?"

"It doesn't seem to be—uh, typical."

"Faulty observation," Wolfe snapped. "Or a defect in your training. Specifically, it's a persecution complex."

"Who's doing the persecuting?"

Wolfe shut his eyes. "I feel it coming on again. Tell him, Archie."

I met Vollmer's gaze. "Look, Doc, the situation is serious. As you know, he was investigating the Boone-Gunther murders for the NIA. The high command didn't like the way Inspector Cramer was handling it and booted him, and replaced him with a baboon by the name of Ash."

"I know. It was in the evening paper."

"Yeah. In tomorrow's evening paper you'll learn that Nero Wolfe has returned the NIA retainer and quit."

"For God's sake, why?"

"I'm telling you. Ash's personal attitude toward Wolfe is such that he would rather slice his wrists than slash his throat because it would prolong the agony. Today he got a material witness warrant and Wolfe had to go to Centre Street, me taking him. Hombert had the warrant killed, for various reasons, but the main one was that Wolfe was working for the NIA, and if the NIA gets offended any worse than it is now it will probably fire the Mayor and everyone else and declare New York a monarchy. But. Wolfe no sooner gets home than he breaks off relations with the NIA. They'll get his letter, with check enclosed, in the morning mail. Whereupon hell will pop wide open. What the NIA will do we don't know and maybe we don't care—I should say maybe Wolfe doesn't care. But we know damn well what the cops will do. First, with Wolfe no longer sleeping with the NIA, that motive for tenderness will be gone. Second, they know that Wolfe has never yet had a murderer for a client, and they know what a job it is to pry him loose from money, especially thirty thousand bucks and up, and they will therefore deduce that one of the NIA boys is guilty, and that Wolfe knows it and knows who it is."

"Who is it?"

I shook my head. "I don't know, and since Wolfe's a raving lunatic you can't ask him. With that setup, it's a cinch to read the future. The wagon will be at the door ready for him, with the papers all in order, any time after ten o'clock, possibly earlier. It's a shame to disappoint them, but all I can do is meet them with another kind of paper, signed by a reputable physician, certifying that in Wolfe's present condition it would be dangerous either to move him from his bed or to permit anyone to converse with him."

I waved a hand. "That's how it stands. Five years ago, the time Wolfe did you a little favor when that crook—what was his name? Griffin—tried to frame you on a malpractice suit, and you told Wolfe if he ever wanted anything all he had to do was ask for it, I warned you you might regret it some day. Brother, this is the day."

Vollmer was rubbing his chin. He didn't really look reluctant, merely thoughtful. He looked at Wolfe, saying nothing, and then returned to me and spoke:

"Naturally I have an uncontrollable itch to ask a lot of questions. This is absolutely fascinating. I suppose the questions wouldn't be answered?"

"I'm afraid not. Not by me anyhow, because I don't know the answers. You might try the patient."

"How long will the certificate have to function?"

"I have no idea. Damn it, I tell you I'm ignorant."

"If he's bad enough to prohibit visitors I'll have to insist on calling on him at least twice a day. And to make it good there ought to be nurses."

"No," I said firmly. "I grant there ought to be, but he would run a fever. Nurses are out. As for you, call as often as you want to. I may get lonely. And make that certificate as strong as they come. Say it would kill him if anybody whose name begins with A even looked at him."

"It will be so worded as to serve its purpose. I'll bring it over in ten minutes or so." Vollmer stood up with his toolbox in his hand. "I did say that time, though, that Wolfe would get anything *he* asked for." He looked at Wolfe. "It would be gratifying just to hear you ask me for something. How about it?"

Wolfe groaned. "They come in hordes," he said distinctly, but in a phony voice. "In chariots with spiked wheels, waving the insolent banners of inflation! Five dollars for a pound of corned beef! Ten dollars for a squab! Sixty cents—"

"I'd better be going," Vollmer said, and moved.

32.

I DIDN'T get lonely during the two and a half days—Thursday, Friday, and part of Saturday—that the certificate worked. Newspapermen, cops, FBI's, NIA's—they all appreciated that I was holding the fort under trying circumstances and did their best to keep my mind occupied so I wouldn't fret. If ordinarily I earn twice as much as I get, which is a conservative estimate, during those sixty-some hours it was ten times as much at a minimum.

Throughout the siege Wolfe stayed put in his room, with the door locked and one of the keys in my pocket and one in Fritz's. Keeping away from the office, dining room, and kitchen for that length of time was of course a hardship, but the real sacrifice, the one that hurt, was giving up his two-a-day trips to the plant rooms. I had to bully him into it, explaining that if a surprise detachment shoved a search warrant at me I might or might not be able to get him back into bed in time, and besides, Theodore slept out, and while he was no traitor he might inadvertently spill it that his afflicted employer did not seem to be goofy among the orchids. For the same reason I refused to let Theodore come down to the bedroom for consultations. I told Wolfe Thursday or Friday, I forget which:

"You're putting on an act. Okay. Applause. Since it requires you to be out of circulation that leaves it strictly up to me and I make the rules. I am already handicapped enough by not knowing one single goddam thing about what you're up to. We had a—"

"Nonsense," he growled. "You know all about it. I have twenty men looking for that cylinder. Nothing can be done without that cylinder. It must be found and it will be. I simply prefer to wait here in my room instead of in jail."

"Nuts." I was upset because I had just spent a hot half hour with another NIA delegation down in the office. "Why did you have to break with the NIA before you went to bed to wait? Granting that one of them did it and you know all about it, which everybody is now sure of but you'll have to show me, that was no reason to return their money in order to keep from having a murderer for a client, because you said yourself that no man was your client, the NIA was. Why in the name of God did you return their dough? And if this cylinder gag is not merely a stall, if it's really it and all the it there is, as you say, what if it never is found? What are you going to do, stay in bed the rest of your life, with Doc Vollmer renewing the certificate on a monthly basis?"

"It will be found," he said meekly. "It was not destroyed, it exists, and therefore it will be found."

I stared at him suspiciously, shrugged, and beat it. When he gets meek it is absolutely no use. I went back to the office and sat and scowled at the Stenophone machine standing over in a corner. My chief reason for admitting that Wolfe really meant what he said about the cylinder was that we were paying a dollar a day rent for that machine.

Not the only reason, however. Bill Gore and twenty Bascom men were actually looking for the cylinder, no question about it. I had been instructed to read the reports before taking them up to Wolfe, and they were quite a chapter in the history of hunting. Bill Gore and another guy were working on all of Phoebe Gunther's friends and even acquaintances in Washington, and two others were doing likewise in New York. Three were flying all over the country, to places where she knew people, on the theory that she might have mailed the cylinder to one of them, though that seemed like a bum theory if, as Wolfe had said, she had wanted to have it easily accessible on short notice. His figure of a grand a day hadn't been so far out after all. One had learned that she had gone to a beauty parlor that Friday afternoon in New York, and he had turned it inside out. Three had started working on parcel rooms everywhere, but had discovered that parcel rooms were being worked by the police and the FBI, armed with authority, so they had switched to another field. They were trying to find out or guess all the routes she had taken on foot and were spending their days on the sidewalks, keeping their eyes peeled for something, anything—a window box with dirt in it, for instance—where she might have made a cache. The rest of them were trying this and that. Friday evening, to take my mind off my troubles, I tried to figure out some possible spot that they were missing. I kept at it an hour, with no result. They were certainly covering the territory.

There were unquestionably twenty-one expensive men on the cylinder chase, but what stuck in my craw was Saul Panzer. No matter what you had on the program Saul rated star billing, and he was not among the twenty-one at all. As far as I was allowed to know he was not displaying the slightest interest in any cylinder. Every couple of hours he phoned in, I didn't know from where, and I obeyed instructions to connect him with Wolfe's bedside extension and keep off the line. Also he made two personal appearances—one at breakfast time Thursday morning and one late Friday afternoon—and each time he spent a quarter of an hour alone with Wolfe and then departed. By that time I was so damn cylinder-conscious that I was inclined to suspect Saul of being engaged in equipping a factory in a Brooklyn basement so we could roll our own.

As the siege continued, my clashes with Wolfe increased both in frequency and in range. One, Thursday afternoon, concerned Inspector Cramer. Wolfe buzzed me on the house phone and told me he wished to have a telephone conversation with Cramer, so would I please dig him up. I flatly refused. My point was that no matter how bitter Cramer might be, or how intensely he might desire to spray Ash with concentrated DDT, he was still a cop, and was therefore not to be trusted with any evidence, as for instance Wolfe's voice sounding natural and making sense, that would tend to cast doubt on Doc Vollmer's certificate. Wolfe finally settled for my getting the dope on Cramer's whereabouts and availability, and that proved to be easy. Lon Cohen told me he had taken a two weeks' leave of absence, for sulking, and when I dialed the number of Cramer's home he answered the phone himself. He kept the conversation brief and to the point, and when I had hung up I got Wolfe on the house phone and told him:

"Cramer's on leave of absence and is staying home licking his wounds, possibly bedridden. He wouldn't say. Anyhow, he can be reached there any time, but he is not affable. I have a notion to send Doc Vollmer to see him."

"Good. Come up here. I'm having trouble with this window again."

"Damn it, you stay in bed and keep away from the windows!"

One feature of the play was that I was not supposed to deny entry to any legitimate caller. That was to convey the impression that our household was not churlish, far from it, but merely stricken with misfortune. Although newspapermen and various other assorted prospectors kept me hopping, the worst nuisances were the NIA and the cops. Around ten Thursday morning Frank Thomas Erskine phoned. He wanted Wolfe but of course didn't get him. I did my best to make the situation clear, but I might as well have tried to explain to a man dying of thirst that the water was being saved to do the laundry with. Less than an hour later here they came, all six of them—the two Erskines, Winterhoff, Breslow, O'Neill, and Hattie Harding. I was courteous, took them to the office, gave them seats, and told them that a talk with Wolfe was positively not on the agenda.

They seemed to be under the impression, judging from their attitudes and tones, that I was not a fellow being but a cockroach. At times it was a little difficult to keep up with them, because they were all full of ideas and words to express them and no one acted as chairman to grant the floor and prevent overlapping. Their main gripes were, first, that it was an act of treachery and betrayal for Wolfe to return their money; second, that if he did it because he was sick he should have said so in his letter; third, that he should immediately and publicly announce his sickness in order to stop the widespread and growing rumor that he broke with the NIA because he got hold of conclusive evidence that the NIA had committed murder; fourth, that if he did have evidence of an NIA man's guilt they wanted to know who and what it was within five minutes; fifth, that they didn't believe he was sick; sixth, who was the doctor; seventh, if he was sick how soon would he be well; eighth, did I realize that in the two days and three nights that had passed since the second murder, Phoebe Gunther's, the damage to the NIA had become incalculable and irretrievable; ninth, fifty or sixty lawyers were of the opinion that Wolfe's abandoning the case without notice would vastly increase the damage and was therefore actionable; tenth, eleventh and twelfth, and so on.

Through the years I have seen a lot of sore, frantic, and distressed people in that office, but this aggregation of specimens was second to none. As far as I could see the common calamity had united them again and the danger of an indiscriminate framing bee had been averted. At one point their unanimous longing to confront Wolfe reached such proportions that Breslow, O'Neill, and young Erskine actually made for the stairs and started up, but when I yelled after them, above the uproar, that the door was locked and if they busted it in Wolfe would probably shoot them dead, they faltered, about-faced, and came back for some more of me.

I made one mistake. Like a simp I told them I would keep a continual eye on Wolfe on the chance of his having a lucid interval, and if one arrived and the doctor permitted I would notify Erskine and he could saddle up and gallop down for an interview. I should have foreseen that not only would they keep the phone humming day and night to ask how about some lucidity, but also they would take turns appearing in person, in singles, pairs, and trios, to sit in the office and wait for some. Which they did. Friday some of them were there half the time, and Saturday morning they started in again. As far as their damn money was concerned, I did at least thirty thousand dollars' worth of entertaining.

After their first visit, Thursday morning, I went up and reported in full to Wolfe, adding that I had not seen fit to inform them that he was keeping the cylinder hounds on the job at his own expense. Wolfe only muttered:

"It doesn't matter. They'll learn it when the time comes."

"Yeah. The scientific name for the disease you've got is acute malignant optimism."

As for the cops, I was instructed by Wolfe to try to prevent an avalanche by volunteering information without delay, and therefore had phoned the Commissioner's office at eight-thirty Thursday morning, before any mail could have been opened up at the NIA office. Hombert hadn't arrived yet, nor had his secretary, but I described the situation to some gook and asked him to pass it on. An hour later Hombert himself called, and the conversation was almost verbatim what it would have been if I had written it down before it took place. He said he was sorry Wolfe had collapsed under the strain, and that the police official who would shortly be calling to see him would be instructed to conduct himself diplomatically and considerately. When I explained that it was doctor's orders that no one at all should see him, not even an insurance salesman, Hombert got brusque and wanted Vollmer's full name and address, which I obligingly furnished. He wanted to know if I had told the press that Wolfe was off the case, and I said no, and he said his office would attend to that to make sure they got it straight. Then he said that Wolfe's action, dropping his client, put it beyond argument that he knew the identity of the murderer, and was probably in possession of evidence against him, and since I was Wolfe's confidential assistant it was to be presumed that I shared the knowledge and the possession, and I was of course aware of the personal risk incurred by failing to communicate such information to the police immediately. I satisfied him on that point, I don't think. Anyhow I was telling the truth, and since I'm not very good at telling the truth I couldn't very well expect him to believe me.

In less than half an hour Lieutenant Rowcliffe and a detective sergeant showed up and I conducted them into the office. Rowcliffe read Doc Vollmer's certificate thoroughly, three times, and I offered to type a copy for him to take along for further study. He was keeping himself under restraint, since it was obvious that thunder and lightning would be wasted. He tried to insist that it wouldn't hurt a bit for him to tiptoe into Wolfe's room just for a compassionate look at a prostrated fellow citizen, and indeed a professional colleague, but I explained that much as the idea appealed to me I didn't dare because Doc Vollmer would never forgive me. He said he understood my position perfectly, and how about my getting wise to myself and spilling some beans? I was, I told him, fresh out of beans. He came about as close to believing me as Hombert had, but there was nothing he could do about it short of taking me downtown and using a piece of hose on me, and Rowcliffe knew me almost as well as he disliked me, so that didn't strike him as feasible.

When they departed Rowcliffe climbed in the police car and rolled away, and the sergeant began strolling up and down the sidewalk in front of the house. That was sensible. There was no point in hiring a window across the street or some similar subtlety, since they knew that we knew there would be a constant eye on our door. From there on we had a sentry out front right up to the end.

I never did understand why they didn't try quicker and harder to break it up, but I suspect it was on account of friction between Inspector Ash and the high command. Later, after it was all over, I tried to find out from Purley Stebbins what had gone on, but Purley never was willing to contribute more than a couple of grunts, probably because the Ash regime was something he wanted to erase from memory. Doc Vollmer got more of it than I did. He kept me informed when he came to pay visits to his patient. The first one, Thursday morning, I escorted him up to the bedroom, but when Wolfe started to enjoy himself by pointing a shaking finger at the wall and declaring that big black worms covered with dollar signs were crawling down from the ceiling, we both got out of there. Thereafter Vollmer never went near the patient, merely staying in the office chinning with me long enough to make it a call for the benefit of the sidewalk sentry. The police were pestering him, but he was getting a kick out of it. Thursday morning Rowcliffe had called on him right after leaving me, and that afternoon a police doctor had come to his office to get information about Wolfe on a professional level. Friday morning Ash himself had showed up, and twenty minutes with Ash had made Vollmer more enthusiastic than ever about the favor he was doing Wolfe. Later Friday afternoon another police doctor had come and had put Vollmer over some high hurdles. When Vollmer dropped in that evening he was, for the first time, not complctely cocky about it.

Saturday noon the blow fell—the one I had been expecting ever since the charade started, and the one Vollmer was leery about. It landed via the telephone, a call from Rowcliffe at twenty past twelve. I was alone in the office when the bell rang, and I was even more alone when it was over and I hung up. I took the stairs two at a time, unlocked Wolfe's door, entered, and announced:

"Okay, Pagliaccio, luck is with us at last. You are booked for the big time. An eminent neurologist named Green, hired by the City of New York and equipped with a court order, will arrive to give you an audition at a quarter to six." I glared down at him and demanded, "Now what? If you try to bull it through I resign as of sixteen minutes to six."

"So." Wolfe closed his book with a finger in it. "This is what we've been fearing." He made the book do the split on the black coverlet. "Why must it be today? Why the devil did you agree on an hour?"

"Because I had to! Who do you think I am, Joshua? They wanted to make it right now, and I di[illegible]e best I could. I told them your doctor had to be present and he couldn't make it until after dinner this evening, nine o'clock. They said it had to be before six o'clock and they wouldn't take no. Damn it, I got an extra five hours and I had to fight for it!"

"Quit yelling at me." His head went back to the pillow. "Go back downstairs. I'm going to have to think."

I stood my ground. "Do you actually mean you haven't

got it figured out what to do? When I've warned you it would come any minute ever since Thursday morning?"

"Archie. Get out of here. How can I put my mind on it with you standing there bellowing?"

"Very well. I'll be in the office. Call me when you get around to it."

I went out, shut the door and locked it, and descended. In the office the phone was ringing. It was only Winterhoff, inquiring after my employer's health.

33.

I TRY, as I go along, not to leave anything essential out of this record, and, since I'm telling it, I regard my own state of mind at various stages as one of the essentials. But for that two hours on Saturday, from twelve-thirty to two-thirty, my state of mind was really not fit to be recorded for family reading. I have a vague recollection that I ate lunch twice, though Fritz politely insists that he doesn't remember it that way. He says that Wolfe's lunch was completely normal as far as he knows—tray taken upstairs full at one o'clock and brought down empty an hour later—and that nothing struck him as abnormal except that Wolfe was too preoccupied to compliment him on the omelet.

What made me use up a month's supply of profanity in a measly two hours was not that all I could see ahead was ignominious surrender. That was a hard dose but by no means fatal. The hell of it was, as I saw it, that we were being bombed out of a position that no one but a maniac would ever have occupied in the first place. I had a right to assume, now that I was reading the reports from Bill Gore and Bascom's men, that I knew exactly what was going on in every sector except the one that was occupied by Saul Panzer, and it was impossible to imagine what Saul could be doing that could justify, let alone necessitate, the gaudy and spectacular stunt Wolfe was indulging in. When Saul phoned in at two o'clock I had a notion to tackle him and try to open him up, but I knew it would be hopeless and put him through to the bedroom. On any list of temptations I have resisted, that one goes first. I was tingling from head to foot with the desire to listen in. But a part of the understanding between Wolfe and me is that I never violate instructions except when circumstances unknown to him, as interpreted by my best judgment, require it, and I couldn't kid myself that that applied here. My instructions were that Saul Panzer was out of bounds for me until further notice, and I put the thing on the cradle and walked up and down with my hands in my pockets.

Other phone calls came, it doesn't matter what, and I did violate another instruction, the one to receive any and all callers. Circumstances certainly justified that. I was in the kitchen helping Fritz sharpen knives, I suppose on the principle that in times of crisis we instinctively seek the companionship of fellow creatures, when the bell rang and I went to the front door, fingered the curtain aside for a peek, and saw Breslow. I opened the door a crack and barked through at him:

"No admittance this is a house of mourning beat it!"

I banged the door and started back to the kitchen, but didn't make it. Passing the foot of the stairs I became aware of sound and movement, and stopping to look up I saw what was making it. Wolfe, covered with nothing but the eight yards of yellow silk it took to make him a suit of pajamas, was descending. I goggled at him. If nothing else, it was unprecedented for him to move vertically except with the elevator.

"How did you get out?" I demanded.

"Fritz gave me a key." He came on down, and I noted that at least he had put his slippers on. He commanded me, "Get Fritz and Theodore in the office at once."

I had never before seen him outside his room in deshabille. It was obviously an extreme emergency. I swung the kitchen door open and spoke to Fritz and then went to the office, buzzed the plant rooms on the house phone, and told Theodore to make it snappy. By the time Theodore trotted down and in, Wolfe was seated behind his desk and Fritz and I were standing by.

"How are you, Theodore? I haven't seen you for three days."

"I'm all right, thank you, sir. I've missed you."

"No doubt." Wolfe's glance went from him to Fritz, then to me, and he said slowly and clearly, "I am a brainless booby."

"Yes, sir," I said cordially.

He frowned. "So are you, Archie. Neither of us has any right, henceforth, to pretend possession of the mental processes of an anthropoid. I include you because you heard what I said to Mr. Hombert and Mr. Skinner. You have read the reports from Mr. Bascom's men. You know what's going on. And by heaven, it hasn't occurred to you that Miss Gunther was alone in this office for a good three minutes, nearer four or five, when you brought her here that evening! And it occurred to me only just now! Pfui! And I have dared for nearly thirty years to exercise my right to vote!" He snorted. "I have the brain of a mollusk!"

"Yeah." I was staring at him. I remembered, of course, that when I had brought Phoebe that Friday night I had left her in the office and gone to the kitchen to get him. "So you think—"

"No. I am through pretending to think. This makes it untenable. —Fritz and Theodore, a young woman was in here alone four minutes. She had, in her pocket or her bag, an object she wanted to hide—a black cylinder three inches in diameter and six inches long. She didn't know how much time she would have; someone might enter any moment. On the assumption that she hid it in this room, find it. Knowing the quality of her mind, I think it likely that she hid it in my desk. I'll look there myself."

He shoved his chair back and dived to pull open a bottom drawer. I was at my own desk, also opening drawers. Fritz asked me, "What do we do, divide it in sections?"

"Divide hell," I told him over my shoulder. "Just start looking."

Fritz went to the couch and began removing cushions. Theodore chose, for his first guess, the two vases on top of the filing cabinet which at that season contained pussy willows. There was no more conversation; we were too busy. I can't give a detailed report of the part of the search conducted by Fritz and Theodore because I was too intent on my own part of it; all I had for them was occasional glances to see what they were covering; but I kept an eye on Wolfe because I shared his opinion of the quality of Phoebe's mind and it would have been like her to pick Wolfe's own desk for it provided she found a drawer which looked as if its contents were not often disturbed. But he drew a blank. As I was opening the back of the radio cabinet, which could be got at without moving the cabinet, he slid his chair back into position, got comfortable in it, muttered, "Confound that woman," and surveyed us like a field commander directing his troops in action.

Fritz's voice came, "Is this it, Mr. Wolfe?"

He was kneeling on the rug in front of the longest section of bookshelves, and stacked beside him were a dozen volumes of the bound *Lindenia,* with a big gap showing on the bottom shelf, which was only a few inches above the floor. He was extending a hand with an object in it at which one glance was enough.

"Ideal," Wolfe said approvingly. "She was really extraordinary. Give it to Archie. Archie, roll that machine out. Theodore, I'll be with you in the potting room possibly later today, certainly tomorrow morning at the usual hour. Fritz, I congratulate you; you tried the bottom shelf first, which was sensible."

Fritz was beaming as he handed me the cylinder and turned to go, with Theodore following him.

"Well," I remarked as I plugged the machine in and inserted the cylinder, "this may do it. Or it may not."

"Start it," Wolfe growled. He was tapping on an arm of his chair with a finger. "What's the matter? Won't it go?"

"Certainly it will go. Don't hurry me. I'm nervous and I have the brain of a—I forget what. Mollusk."

I flipped the switch and sat down. The voice of Cheney Boone came to our ears, unmistakably the same voice we had heard on the other ten cylinders. For five minutes neither of us moved a muscle. I stared at the grill of the loud-speaker attachment, and Wolfe leaned back with his eyes closed. When it came to the end I reached and turned the switch.

Wolfe sighed clear to the bottom, opened his eyes, and straightened up.

"Our literature needs some revision," he declared. "For example, 'dead men tell no tales.' Mr. Boone is dead. Mr. Boone is silent. But he speaks."

"Yep." I grinned at him. "The silent speaker. Science is wonderful, but I know one guy who won't think so, goddam him. Shall I go get him?"

"No. We can arrange this, I think, by telephone. You have Mr. Cramer's number?"

"Sure."

"Good. But first get Saul. You'll find him at Manhattan five, three-two-three-two."

34.

By ten minutes to four our guests had all arrived and were collected in the office. One of them was an old friend and enemy: Inspector Cramer. One was an ex-client: Don O'Neill. One was merely a recent acquaintance: Alger Kates. The fourth was a complete stranger: Henry A. Warder, Vice-President and Treasurer of O'Neill and Warder, Incorporated. Don O'Neill's vice. Saul Panzer, who had retired to a chair over in the corner behind the globe, was of course not regarded as a guest but as one of the family.

Cramer was in the red leather chair, watching Wolfe like a hawk. O'Neill, entering and catching sight of his Vice-President, who had arrived before him, had immediately hit the ceiling, and then had just as immediately thought better of it, clamped his mouth shut, and congealed. The vice, Henry A. Warder, who was both broad and tall, built like a concrete buttress, looked as if he could use some buttressing himself. He was the only one whose demeanor suggested that smelling salts might be called for, being obviously scared silly. Alger Kates had not spoken a word to anyone, not a word, not even when I let him in. His basic attitude was that of a Sunday School teacher in a den of thieves.

Wolfe had clothes on for the first time since Wednesday evening. He sat and did a circle with his eyes, taking them in, and spoke:

"This is going to be disagreeable, gentlemen, for all three of you, so let's make it as brief as we can. I'll do my share. The quickest way is to begin by letting you listen to a Stenophone cylinder, but first I must tell you where I got it. It was found in this room an hour ago, behind the books"—he pointed—"on that bottom shelf. Miss Gunther placed it there, hid it there, when she came to see me Friday evening a week ago—a week ago last evening."

"She wasn't here," O'Neill rasped. "She didn't come."

Wolfe regarded him without affection. "So you don't want this to be brief."

"You're damn right I do! The briefer the better!"

"Then don't interrupt. Naturally everything I'm saying is not only true but provable, or I wouldn't be saying it. Miss Gunther came that evening, brought by Mr. Goodwin, after the others left, and happened to be alone in this room for several minutes. That I did not remember that sooner and search the room was inexcusable. It was an appalling failure of an intellect which has sometimes been known to function satisfactorily.

"However." He made a brusque gesture. "That is between me and the universe. We shall now listen to that cylinder, which was dictated by Mr. Boone his last afternoon at his office in Washington. Do not, I beg you, interrupt it. Archie, turn it on."

There were murmurs as I flipped the switch. Then Cheney Boone, the silent speaker, had the floor:

> Miss Gunther, this is for no one but you and me. Make sure of that. One carbon only, for your locked file, and deliver the original to me.
>
> I have just had a talk in a hotel room with Henry A.

> Warder, Vice-President and Treasurer of O'Neill and Warder. He is the man who has been trying to reach me through you and refusing to give his name. He finally got me directly, at home, and I made this appointment with him, for today, March 26th. He told me the following—

Warder catapulted out of his chair and started for the machine, screaming, "Stop it!"

It would be more in keeping with his size and appearance to say that he roared or blared, but it literally was a scream. Having anticipated some such demonstration, I had placed the machine at the end of my desk, only four feet from me, and therefore had no difficulty intercepting the attack. I planted myself in Warder's line of approach, reached back of me to turn the switch, and spoke firmly:

"Nothing stirring. Back up and sit down." From my coat pocket I produced an automatic and let it be seen. "All three of you are going to like it less and less as it goes along. If you get a simultaneous idea and try to act on it, I'll wing you and it will be a pleasure."

"That was under a pledge of confidence!" Warder was trembling from head to foot. "Boone promised—"

"Can it!" Cramer had left his chair and was beside Warder. He asked me, "They haven't been gone over, have they?"

"They're not gunmen," Wolfe snapped. "They merely club people on the head—or one of them does."

Cramer paid no attention to him. He started with Warder, gave him a quick but thorough frisking, motioned him back, and said to O'Neill, "Stand up." O'Neill didn't move. Cramer barked at him, "Do you want to get lifted?" O'Neill stood up and did some fancy breathing while Cramer's expert hands went over him. When it was Alger Kates's turn no pressure was required. He looked dazed but not even resentful. Cramer, through with him and empty-handed, moved across to the machine and stood with a hand resting on its frame. He growled at me:

"Go ahead, Goodwin."

Not being a Stenophone expert and not wanting to damage the cylinder, I started it over at the beginning. Soon it was at the point where it had been interrupted:

> He told me the following. Warder has known for several months that the president of his company, Don O'Neill, has been paying a member of the BPR staff for confidential information. He did not discover it by accident or any secret investigation. O'Neill has not only admitted it, but bragged about it, and Warder, as Treasurer,

has been obliged to supply corporation funds for the purpose through a special account. He has done so under protest. I repeat that this is Warder's story, but I am inclined to believe it as he tells it because he came to me voluntarily. It will have to be checked with the FBI to find out if they have had any lead in the direction of O'Neill and Warder and specifically Warder, but the FBI must not be given any hint of Warder's communicating with me. I had to give him my pledge on that before he would say a word, and the pledge must be kept absolutely. I'll talk this over with you tomorrow, but I have a hunch—you know how I have hunches—that I want to get it on a cylinder without delay.

Cramer made a little noise that was part snort and part sneeze, and three pairs of eyes went to him as if in irritation at his interfering with a fascinating performance. I didn't mind so much because I had heard it before. What I was interested in was the audience.

Warder said that to his knowledge the payments began last September and that the total paid to date is sixteen thousand five hundred dollars. The reason he gave for coming to me is that he is a man of principle, so he put it, and he violently disapproves of bribery, especially bribery of government officials. He was not in a position to take a firm stand with O'Neill because O'Neill owns over sixty per cent of the corporation's stock and Warder owns less than ten per cent, and O'Neill could and would throw him out. That can easily be checked. Warder was extremely nervous and apprehensive. My impression is that his story is straight, that his coming to me was the result of his conscience gnawing at him, but there is a chance that his real motive is to build a fire under O'Neill, for undisclosed reasons. He swore that his only purpose was to acquaint me with the facts so I can put a stop to it by getting rid of my corrupted subordinate, and that is substantiated by his exacting a pledge beforehand that makes it impossible for us to touch O'Neill in the matter.

This will be a surprise to you—I know it was to me—the man O'Neill has bought is Kates, Alger Kates. You know what I have thought of Kates, and, so far as I know, you have thought the same. Warder claims he doesn't know exactly what O'Neill has got for his money, but that isn't important. We know what Kates has been in a position to sell—as much as any man in the organization outside of the very top ranks—and our only safe assumption is that he has given it all to O'Neill and that O'Neill has passed it on to the whole rotten NIA gang. I don't need to tell you how sick I am about it. For a miserable sixteen thousand dollars. I don't think I would mind quite so much being betrayed by a first-class snake for something up in the millions, but this just makes me sick. I thought Kates was a modest little man with his heart in his work and in our objectives and purposes. I have no idea what he wanted the money for and I don't care. I haven't decided how to handle it. The best way would be to put the FBI on him and catch him with O'Neill, but I don't know whether my pledge to Warder would permit that. I'll think it over and we'll discuss it tomorrow. If I were face to face with Kates right now I don't think I could control myself. Actually I don't ever want to see him again. This has gone pretty deep and if he entered this room now I think I'd get my fingers around his throat and choke him to death. You know me. That's the way I talk.

The important thing is not Kates himself, but what this shows. It shows that it is simply insanity for me to put complete trust in anybody, anyone whatever except Dexter and you, and we must install a much better system of checks immediately. To some extent we can continue to let the FBI handle it, but we must reinforce that with a setup and personnel that will work directly under us. I want you to think it over for tomorrow's discussion, to which no one will be invited but Dexter. The way it strikes me now, you'll have to take this over and drop everything else. That will leave me in a hole, but this is vitally important. Think it over. I have to appear before the Senate Committee in the morning, so I'll take this to New York and give it to you, and you can run it off while I'm up on the Hill, and we'll get at it as early in the afternoon as possible.

The voice stopped and was replaced by a faint sizzling purr, and I reached to flip the switch.

There was complete dead silence.

Wolfe broke it. "What about it, Mr. Kates?" he asked in a tone of innocent curiosity. "When you entered that room, taking Mr. Boone material for his speech, and he found himself face to face with you, did he get his fingers around your throat and try to choke you?"

"No," Kates squeaked. He sounded indignant, but that may have been only because squeaks often do.

O'Neill commanded him: "You keep out of this, Kates! Keep your mouth shut!"

Wolfe chuckled. "That's marvelous, Mr. O'Neill. It really is. Almost verbatim. That first evening here you admonished him, word for word, 'You can keep out of this, Kates! Sit down and shut up!' It was not very intelligent of you, since it sounded precisely like a high-handed man ordering an employee around, as indeed it was. It led to my having a good man spend three days trying to find a link between you and Mr. Kates, but you had been too circumspect." His eyes darted back to Kates. "I asked about Mr. Boone's choking you because apparently he had it in mind, and also because it suggests a possible line for you—self-defense. A good lawyer might do something with it—but then of course there's Miss Gunther. I doubt if a jury could be persuaded that she too tried to choke you, there on my stoop. By the way, there's one detail I'm curious about. Miss Gunther told Mrs. Boone that she wrote a letter to the murderer, telling him that he must return that wedding picture. I don't believe it. I don't think Miss Gunther would have put anything like that in writing. I think she got the picture and the automobile license from you and mailed them to Mrs. Boone herself. Didn't she?"

For reply Alger Kates put on one of the strangest performances I have ever seen, and I have seen plenty. He squeaked, and this time there was no question about the indignation, not at Wolfe but at Inspector Cramer. He was trembling with indignation, up on his feet, a retake in every way of the dramatic moment when he had accused Breslow of going beyond the bounds of common decency. He squeaked, "The police were utterly incompetent! They should have found out where that piece of pipe came from in a few hours! They never did! It came from a pile of rubbish in a basement hall in the building on Forty-first Street where the NIA offices are!"

"For Christ's sake," Cramer rumbled. "Listen to him! He's sore!"

"He's a fool," O'Neill said righteously, apparently addressing the Stenophone. "He's a contemptible fool. I certainly never suspected him of murder." He turned to look straight at Kates. "Good God, I never thought you were capable of that!"

"Neither did I," Kates squeaked. He had stopped trembling and was standing straight, holding himself stiff. "Not before it happened. After it happened I understood myself better. I wasn't as much of a fool as Phoebe was. She should have known it then, what I was capable of. I did. She wouldn't even promise not to tell or to destroy that cylinder. She wouldn't even promise!" He kept his unblinking eyes on O'Neill. "I should have killed you too, that same evening. I could have. You were afraid of me. You're afraid of me right now! Neither of them was afraid of me, but you are! You say you never suspected me of murder when you knew all about it!"

O'Neill started a remark, but Cramer squelched him and asked Kates, "How did he know all about it?"

"I told him." If Kates's squeak was as painful to perform as it was to listen to he was certainly being hurt. "Or rather I didn't have to tell him. He arranged to meet me—"

"That's a lie," O'Neill said coldly and precisely. "Now you're lying."

"Okay, let him finish it." Cramer kept at Kates, "When was that?"

"The next day, Wednesday. Wednesday afternoon. We met that evening."

"Where?"

"On Second Avenue between Fifty-third and Fifty-fourth. We talked there on the sidewalk. He gave me some money and told me that if anything happened, if I was arrested, he would furnish whatever I needed. He was afraid of me then. He kept watching me, watching my hands."

"How long were you together?"

"Ten minutes. My estimate would be ten minutes."

"What time was it?"

"Ten o'clock. We were to meet at ten o'clock and I was on time, but he was late about fifteen minutes because he said he had to make sure he wasn't being followed. I don't think an intelligent man should have any trouble about that."

Wolfe broke in. "Mr. Cramer. Isn't this a waste of time? You're going to have to go all over it again downtown, with a stenographer. He seems to be ready to co-operate."

"He is ready," O'Neill put in, "to get himself electrocuted and to make all the trouble he can for other people with his damn lies."

"I wouldn't worry too much about that if I were you." Wolfe regarded O'Neill with a glint in his eyes. "He is at least more of a philosopher than you are. Bad as he is, he has the grace to accept the inevitable with a show of decorum. You, on the contrary, try to wiggle. From the glances you have been directing at Mr. Warder, I suspect you have no clear idea of where you're at. You should be making up with him. You're going to need him to look after the business while you're away."

"I'm seeing this through. I'm not going away."

"Oh, but you are. You're going to jail. At least that

seems—" Wolfe turned abruptly to the Vice-President. "What about it, Mr. Warder? Are you going to try to discredit this message from the dead? Are you going to repudiate or distort your interview with Mr. Boone and have a jury vote you a liar? Or are you going to show that you have some sense?"

Warder no longer looked scared, and when he spoke he showed no inclination to scream. "I am going," he said in a firm and virtuous voice, "to tell the truth."

"Did Mr. Boone tell the truth on that cylinder?"

"Yes. He did."

Wolfe's eyes flashed back to O'Neill. "There you are, sir. Bribery is a felony. You're going to need Mr. Warder. The other matter, complicity in murder as an accessory after the fact—that all depends, mostly on your lawyer. From here on the lawyers take over. —Mr. Cramer. Get them out of here, won't you? I'm tired of looking at them." He shifted to me. "Archie, pack up that cylinder. Mr. Cramer will want to take it along."

Cramer, moving, addressed me: "Hold it, Goodwin, while I use the phone," so I sat facing the audience, with the automatic in my hand in case someone had an attack of nerves, while he dialed his number and conversed. I was interested to hear that his objective was not the Homicide Squad office, where Ash had been installed, nor even the Chief Inspector, but Hombert himself. Cramer did occasionally show signs of having more brain than a mollusk.

"Commissioner Hombert? Inspector Cramer. Yes, sir. No, I'm calling from Nero Wolfe's office. No, sir, I'm not trying to horn in, but if you'll let me . . . Yes, sir, I'm quite aware it would be a breach of discipline, but if you'll just listen a minute—certainly I'm here with Wolfe, I didn't break in, and I've got the man, I've got the evidence, and I've got a confession. That's exactly what I'm telling you, and I'm neither drunk nor crazy. Send—wait a minute, hold it."

Wolfe was making frantic gestures.

"What do you want?" Cramer growled.

"Tell him," Wolfe commanded, "to keep that confounded doctor away from here."

Cramer resumed. "All right, Commissioner. Send up—oh, nothing, just Wolfe raving something about a doctor. Were you sending him a doctor? He don't need one and in my opinion never will. Send three cars and six men to Wolfe's address. No, I don't, but I'm bringing three of them down. You'll see when I get there. Yes, sir, I'm telling you, the case is finished, all sewed up and no gaps worth mentioning. Sure, I'll bring them straight to you. . . ."

He hung up.

"You won't have to put handcuffs on me, will you?" Alger Kates squeaked.

"I want to phone my lawyer," O'Neill said in a frozen voice.

Warder just sat.

35.

SKIPPING a thousand or so minor details over the weekend, such as the eminent neurologist Green—no one having bothered to stop him—showing up promptly at a quarter to six, only a few minutes after Cramer had left with his catch, and being informed, in spite of his court order, that the deal was off, I bounce to Monday morning. Wolfe, coming down from the plant rooms at eleven o'clock, knew that he would have a visitor, Cramer having phoned for an appointment, and when he entered the office the Inspector was there in the red leather chair. Beside him on the floor was a misshapen object covered with green florist's paper which he had refused to let me relieve him of. After greetings had been exchanged and Wolfe had got himself comfortable, Cramer said he supposed that Wolfe had seen in the paper that Kates had signed a full and detailed confession to both murders.

Wolfe nodded. "A foolish and inadequate man, that Mr. Kates. But not intellectually to be despised. One item of his performance might even be called brilliant."

"Sure. I would say more than one. Do you mean his leaving that scarf in his own pocket instead of slipping it into somebody else's?"

"Yes, sir. That was noteworthy."

"He's noteworthy all right," Cramer agreed. "In fact he's in a class by himself. There was one thing he wouldn't talk about or sign any statement about, and what do you suppose it was, something that would help put him in the chair? Nope. We couldn't get anything out of him about what he wanted the money for, and when we asked if it was his wife, trips to Florida and so forth, he stuck his chin out and said as if we was worms, 'We'll leave my wife out of this, you will not mention my wife again.' She got here yesterday afternoon and he won't see her. I think he thinks she's too holy to be dragged in."

"Indeed."

"Indeed yes. But on the part that will do for him he was

perfectly willing to oblige. For instance, with Boone there at the hotel. He entered the room and handed Boone some papers, and Boone threw it at him, what he had found out, and then told him to beat it and turned his back on him, and Kates picked up the monkey wrench and gave it to him. Kates tells us exactly what Boone said and what he said, and then carefully reads it over to be sure we got it down right. The same way with Phoebe Gunther here on your stoop. He wants the story straight. He wants it distinctly understood that he didn't arrange to meet her and come here with her, when she phoned him, he merely waited in an areaway across the street until he saw her coming and then joined her and mounted the stoop with her. The pipe was up his sleeve with the scarf already wrapped around it. Three days before that, the first time they were here, when he swiped the scarf out of Winterhoff's pocket, he didn't know then what he would be using it for, he only thought there might be some way of planting it somewhere to involve Winterhoff—an NIA man."

"Naturally." Wolfe was contributing to the conversation just to be polite. "Anything to keep eyes away from him. Wasted effort, since my eye was already on him."

"It was?" Cramer sounded skeptical. "What put it there?"

"Mostly two things. First, of course, that command Mr. O'Neill gave him here Friday evening, indubitably a command to one from whom he had reason to expect obedience. Second, and much more important, the wedding picture mailed to Mrs. Boone. Granted that there are men capable of that gesture, assuredly none of the five NIA men whom I had met had it in them. Miss Harding was obviously too cold-blooded to indulge in any such act of grace. Mr. Dexter's alibi had been tested and stood. Mrs. Boone and her niece were manifestly not too suspected, not by me. There remained only Miss Gunther and Mr. Kates. Miss Gunther might conceivably have killed Mr. Boone, but not herself with a piece of pipe; and she was the only one of them who could without painful strain on probability be considered responsible for the return of the wedding picture. Then where did she get it? From the murderer. By name, from whom? As a logical and workable conjecture, Mr. Kates."

Wolfe fluttered a hand. "All that was mere phantom-chasing. What was needed was evidence—and all the time here it was, on that bookshelf in my office. That, I confess, is a bitter pill to swallow. Will you have some beer?"

"No, thanks, I guess I won't." Cramer seemed to be nervous or uneasy or something. He looked at the clock and slid to the edge of the chair. "I've got to be going. I just dropped in." He elevated to his feet and shook his pants legs down. "I've got a hell of a busy day. I suppose you've heard that I'm back at my desk at Twentieth Street. Inspector Ash has been moved to Richmond. Staten Island."

"Yes, sir. I congratulate you."

"Much obliged. So with me back at the old stand you'll have to continue to watch your step. Try pulling any fast ones and I'll still be on your neck."

"I wouldn't dream of trying to pull a fast one."

"Okay. Just so we understand each other." Cramer started for the door. I called after him:

"Hey, your package!"

He said over his shoulder, barely halting, "Oh, I forgot, that's for you, Wolfe, hope you like it," and was on his way. Judging from the time it took him to get on out and slam the door behind him, he must have double-quicked.

I went over and lifted the package from the floor, put it on Wolfe's desk, and tore the green paper off, exposing the contents to view. The pot was a glazed sickening green. The dirt was just dirt. The plant was in fair condition, but there were only two flowers on it. I stared at it in awe.

"By God," I said when I could speak, "he brought you an orchid."

"Brassocattleya thorntoni," Wolfe purred. "Handsome."

"Nuts," I said realistically. "You've got a thousand better ones. Shall I throw it out?"

"Certainly not. Take it up to Theodore." Wolfe wiggled a finger at me. "Archie. One of your most serious defects is that you have no sentiment."

"No?" I grinned at him. "You'd be surprised. At this very moment one is almost choking me—namely, gratitude for our good luck at having Cramer back, obnoxious as he is. With Ash there life wouldn't have been worth living."

Wolfe snorted. "Luck!"

36.

SOONER or later I had to make it plain to him that I was not a halfwit. I was waiting for a fitting moment, and it came that same day, Monday afternoon, about an hour after lunch, when we received a phone call from Frank Thomas Erskine. He was permitted to speak to Wolfe, and I listened in at my desk.

The gist of it was that a check for one hundred thousand dollars would be mailed to Wolfe that afternoon, which would seem to be enough gist for one little phone call. The rest was just trivial. The NIA deeply appreciated what Wolfe had done for it and was utterly unable to understand why he had returned its money. It was paying him the full amount of the reward at once, as offered in its advertisement, in advance of the fulfillment of the specified conditions, because of its gratitude and its confidence in him, and also because Kates's signed confession made the fulfillment of the conditions inevitable. It would be glad to pay an additional amount for expenses incurred if Wolfe would say how much. It had discussed the matter with Inspector Cramer, and Cramer had disavowed any claim to any part of the reward and insisted that it all belonged to Wolfe.

It was a nice phone call.

Wolfe said to me with a smirk, "That's satisfactory and businesslike. Paying the reward without delay."

I leered at him. "Yeah? Little does Mr. Erskine know."

"Little does he know what? What's wrong now?"

I threw one knee over the other and settled back. The time had come. "There are," I stated, "several ways of doing this. One would be to put a hunk of butter in your mouth and see if it melted. I prefer my way, which is just to tell you. Or I should say ask you, since I'll put it in the form of questions, only I'll supply the answers myself."

"What the devil are you talking about?"

"No, the questions originate with me. Number one: when did you find the cylinder? Saturday afternoon, when you waddled in here in your pajamas, belittling your brains? Not a chance. You knew where it was all the time, at least for three or four days. You found it either Tuesday morning, while I was down at Cramer's office being wrung out, or Wednesday while I was up having lunch with Nina Boone. I lean to Tuesday, but I admit it may have been Wednesday."

"You shouldn't," Wolfe murmured, "leave things teetering like that."

"Please don't interrupt me. Number two: why, if you knew where the cylinder was, did you pester Mrs. Boone to tell you? Because you wanted to make sure she *didn't* know. If she had known she might have told the cops before you decided to let loose, and the reward would have gone to her, or anyway not to you. And since Phoebe Gunther had told her a lot she might have told her that too. Also, it was part of your general plan to spread the impression that you didn't know where the cylinder was and would give an arm and several teeth to find it."

"That was actually the impression," Wolfe murmured.

"It was indeed. I could back all this up with various miscellaneous items, for instance your sending for the Stenophone Wednesday morning, which is the chief reason I lean to Tuesday, but let's go on to number three: what was the big idea? When you found the cylinder why didn't you say so? Because you let your personal opinions interfere with your professional actions, which reminds me I must do some reading up on ethics. Because your opinion of the NIA coincides roughly with some other people's, including my own, but that's beside the point, and you knew the stink about the murders was raising cain with the NIA, and you wanted to prolong it as much as possible. To accomplish that you even went to the length of letting yourself be locked in your room for three days, but there I admit another factor enters, your love of art for art's sake. You'll do anything to put on a good show, provided you get top billing."

"How long is this going on?"

"I'm about through. Number four, why did you drop the client and return the dough, is easy. There's always a chance that you may change your mind some day and decide you want to go to heaven, and a plain unadulterated double cross would rule it out. So you couldn't very well have kept the NIA's money, and gone on having it for a client, while you were doing your damnedest to push it off a cliff. Here, however, is where I get cynical. What if no reward had been publicly offered? Would you have put on the show just the same? I express no opinion, but boy, I have one. Another thing about ethics—exactly what is the difference between having a client and taking a fee, and accepting a reward?"

"Nonsense. The reward was advertised to a hundred million people and the terms stated. It was to be paid to whoever earned it. I earned it."

"Okay, I merely mention the point. I don't question your going to heaven if you decide you want in. Incidentally, you are not absolutely watertight. If Saul Panzer was put under oath and asked what he did from Wednesday to Saturday, and he replied that he kept in touch with Henry A. Warder to make sure that Warder could be had when needed, and then if you were asked where you got the idea that you might need Henry A. Warder, mightn't you have a little trouble shooting the answer? Not that it will happen, knowing Saul as I do. —Well. Let's see. I guess that's about all. I just wanted you to know that I resent your making contemptuous remarks about your brain."

Wolfe grunted. There was a silence. Then his eyes opened half way and he rumbled:

"You've left one thing out."

"What?"

"A possible secondary motive. Or even a primary one. Taking all that you have said as hypothesis—since of course it is inadmissible as fact—look back at me last Tuesday, six days ago, when—by hypothesis—I found the cylinder. What actually would have taken precedence in my mind?"

"I've been telling you. Not what would have, what did."

"But you left one thing out. Miss Gunther."

"What about her?"

"She was dead. As you know, I detest waste. She had displayed remarkable tenacity, audacity, and even imagination, in using the murder of Mr. Boone for a purpose he would have desired, approved, and applauded. In the middle of it she was herself murdered. Surely she deserved not to have her murder wasted. She deserved to get something out of it. I found myself—by hypothesis—in an ideal position to see that that was taken care of. That's what you left out."

I stared at him. "Then I've got a hypothesis too. If that was it, either primary or secondary, to hell with ethics."

ABOUT THE AUTHOR

REX STOUT, born in Kansas in 1886, has had an extremely varied career. After leaving the Navy in 1908, he became an itinerant bookkeeper and then worked as a sight-seeing guide, bookstore salesman, stablehand, and hotel manager. Later he devised and implemented a school banking system which was installed in four hundred cities and towns throughout the country. In 1927 he retired from the world of finance and began writing. His first Nero Wolfe novel, FER-DE-LANCE, appeared in 1934.

In 1941 Mr. Stout became chairman of the Writer's War Board, and in 1943 he was elected president of the Authors Guild. Since 1946 he has written more than twenty-eight Nero Wolfe books. The most recent titles are THE MOTHER HUNT, TRIO FOR BLUNT INSTRUMENTS, and A RIGHT TO DIE. Mr. Stout lives in Brewster, New York.